PCOS AND GETTING PREGNANT: *A TRIED AND PROVEN STRATEGY TO TREAT PCOS AND BECOME PREGNANT INSTANTLY*

By

Sadie B. Allen

About the Author

Sadie B. Allen is the creative author of " PCOS And Getting Pregnant: A Tried and a Proven Strategy to Treat PCOS and Become Pregnant Instantly" In the realm of women's health, Sadie is a trailblazer, combining her deep understanding of endocrinology with an unwavering dedication to helping individuals who suffer from PCOS. Sadie becomes a trusted advisor for those looking to achieve flourishing health because of her ability to translate complex scientific ideas into practical solutions. She is committed to improving people's lives, as seen by her attempts to demystify PCOS and offer a unique healing process. With her inspiring and caring approach, Sadie is a shining example for anyone seeking long-term wellness while dealing with PC

Abstract

Polycystic Ovarian Syndrome (PCOS) is one of the most common metabolic and reproductive disorders among women of reproductive age. Women suffering from PCOS present with a constellation of symptoms associated with menstrual dysfunction and androgen excess, which significantly impacts their quality of life. They may be at increased risk of multiple morbidities, including obesity, insulin resistance, type II diabetes mellitus, cardiovascular disease (CVD), infertility, cancer, and psychological disorders. This review summarizes what the literature has so far provided from guidelines to diagnosis of PCOS. It will also present a general overview about the morbidities associated with this disease, specifically with its more severe classic form. Finally, the review will stress on the various aspects of treatment and screening recommendations currently used in the management of this condition.

Table of contents

Introduction:

A basic explanation of PCOS

A disorder known as polycystic ovarian syndrome (PCOS) causes the ovaries to overproduce androgens, or male sex hormones, which are typically seen in modest amounts in women. Numerous tiny cysts, or sacs packed with fluid, develop in the ovaries and are referred to as polycystic ovarian syndrome. On the other hand, some women with this disease do not produce cysts, while some women without it do.

Ovulation is the process by which an ovary releases a mature egg. This takes place to enable fertilization by a male sperm. The egg is expelled from the body during your period if it is not fertilized.

Sometimes a woman produces insufficient amounts of the hormones required for ovulation. The ovaries may generate several little cysts if ovulation is unsuccessful. These cysts produce androgens, which are hormones.

High testosterone levels are common in PCOS-affected women. This may result in further issues for a woman's menstrual cycle. Numerous PCOS symptoms may result from it.

Medication is a common treatment for PCOS. While there is no treatment for PCOS, this can help manage symptoms and avoid certain health issues.

What leads to PCOS?

It's unclear what specifically causes PCOS. Insulin resistance is common in female PCOS patients. That indicates poor insulin use by the body. Higher amounts of testosterone may result from the body's accumulation of insulin. Furthermore, obesity might worsen PCOS symptoms by raising insulin levels.

Additionally, PCOS can run in families. Sisters or a mother and daughter are common PCOS cases.

Summary

When your ovaries—the organ that makes and releases eggs—produce too many hormones, it can lead to an imbalance in hormones known as polycystic ovarian syndrome, or PCOS. Your ovaries create an abnormally large amount of androgens when you have PCOS. This throws off the balance of your reproductive hormones. People who have PCOS thus frequently experience irregular menstrual cycles, missed periods, and uncertain ovulation. Due to an ovulation, or the absence of ovulation, small follicular cysts—fluid-filled sacs containing immature eggs—may be seen on your ovaries during an ultrasound. Despite the term "polycystic," PCOS is not necessarily caused by ovarian cysts. The ovarian cysts are not painful or hazardous.

One of the most frequent reasons why women and those who are assigned female at birth (AFAB) experience infertility is PCOS. It may also raise your chance of developing additional medical issues. Depending on your symptoms and if you want to get pregnant, your doctor can treat PCOS.

When does PCOS first manifest?

Every time after puberty, women and people with AFAB can get PCOS. When trying to get pregnant, the majority of people are diagnosed in their 20s or 30s. If you are obese or if other members of your biological family also have PCOS, your chances of developing PCOS may be increased.

How prevalent is PCOS?

PCOS is extremely common; 15% of women and AFAB individuals who are of reproductive age have the condition.

Chapter 1:
PCOS and Conceiving.

What You Should Know About PCOS and Pregnancy-Related Conditions

- Moms' risks
- Risks for a child
- Definition of Conceiving
- Breastfeeding
- Symptoms
- Management
- Next actions

A disorder known as polycystic ovarian syndrome, or PCOS, affects 6–15% of fertile women. It could be more challenging to get pregnant if you have PCOS. Additionally, if you can conceive, there is a chance that your pregnancy, labor, and delivery will be more complicated.

Compared to women without PCOS, women with PCOS have a threefold increased risk of miscarriage. They also have an increased risk of larger babies, early deliveries, gestational diabetes, and preeclampsia. This can cause problems giving birth or necessitate a cesarean section.

Risks for expectant mothers with PCOS

It may be more difficult for you to become pregnant if you have PCOS. An imbalance in hormones could be the cause.

Obesity and reliance on reproductive technologies are associated with PCOS in women. According to one study, 60% of women with PCOS are obese (Trusted sources). To conceive, nearly 14% used reproductive technology.

Women who have PCOS are more likely to experience several health issues throughout their lives, such as:

- Glucose intolerance
- Diabetes type 2
- Elevated cholesterol
- Elevated BP
- Heart conditions
- Heart attack
- Apnea in sleep

Perhaps a higher chance of endometrial cancer

Pregnant women with PCOS are more likely to experience difficulties. Preeclampsia is one such illness that can be harmful to the expectant mother and child. The baby and placenta should be delivered as the prescribed course of treatment to alleviate discomfort. Considering the degree of your symptoms and the gestational age of your unborn child, your doctor will weigh the advantages and disadvantages of delivering your baby at a specific time. If preeclampsia develops during your pregnancy, you will require close monitoring. Gestational diabetes and pregnancy-induced hypertension (high blood pressure) are other issues.

A larger-than-average infant could be the result of gestational diabetes. This can cause issues when the baby is delivered. For instance, shoulder dystopian—a condition in which the baby's shoulder becomes trapped during labor—is more common in larger babies.

With close observation, the majority of PCOS symptoms during pregnancy can be managed. If you get gestational diabetes, you might need to take insulin to keep your blood sugar levels steady.

Risks for a child

Unfortunately, having PCOS while pregnant adds still another level of difficulty. Both you and your child will need to watch it more closely.

Some of the baby's potential PCOS concerns include the following:

- Premature birth
- Enormous given the gestational age
- Loss of pregnancy

- Lowered Apgar score

NOTE: Based on certain studies, your daughter's chances of developing PCOS are 50% higher if she is a girl.

Women with PCOS are also more likely to give birth via cesarean because they tend to have larger-sized kids. It is likely that throughout labor and delivery, new problems will surface.

Pregnancy Resulting From PCOS

Some women may not even be aware that they have PCOS until they try to conceive. PCOS is often disregarded. But if you've been trying for a natural delivery for more than a year, you should talk to your doctor about getting tested.

You can plan your pregnancy with the help of your doctor. Many strategies can increase your chances of getting pregnant, like eating a healthy diet, losing weight, and in certain cases, using medication.

PCOS and breastfeed

If PCOS is diagnosed, you may need to manage symptoms even after getting pregnant. However, there can be variations in the symptoms and intensity. You may need some time to get used to your new "normal" because the symptoms may occasionally vary due to hormonal changes that occur during pregnancy and nursing.

For those with PCOS, breastfeeding is safe—even if you take insulin to help control your blood sugar. For women who have had gestational diabetes, breastfeeding can help lower their chance of developing type 2 diabetes later in life.

If your family feels that nursing is a suitable fit, do your homework, use your resources, and make sure that you and your kid have a positive breastfeeding experience.

Explain PCOS.

PCOS, also known as Stein-Leventhal syndrome, is a hormonal abnormality that primarily affects women. Its defining characteristic is the overproduction of androgens, or "male" hormones.

Women with PCOS may experience acne and excessive hair growth. It can also interfere with regular menstruation cycles and result in ovarian cysts.

The fact that there isn't a single test to identify it makes it a challenging condition. Instead, medical professionals examine the indicators of your body's processes. Signs could include irregular periods or excessive hair growth. Then, medical professionals can piece together a picture of PCOS.

Symptoms of PCOS

Since diagnosing PCOS in women can be challenging, it is frequently overlooked. The symptoms can differ and affect a wide range of women.

For instance, obesity or weight gain may occur often in PCOS patients. It's not a guarantee, though. A lot of PCOS-affected women have slim bodies.

Sadly, up to 50% of women with PCOS never receive a formal diagnosis. This is why PCOS is frequently referred to as the silent killer.

Among the PCOS symptoms that are more prevalent are:

- Cysts called "string of pearls" on the ovaries;
- Insulin resistance;
- Elevated testosterone leading to male pattern baldness,
- Acne, and excessive hair growth;
- Suppressed ovulation;
- Excessive weight gain;
- Weight gain around the midsection
- Dark, thick skin patches on the thighs, arms, breasts, or neck
- Skin tags on the neck or under the armpits

- Pelvic ache
- Depression or anxiety
- Sleep apnea Therapy
- PCOS now has no known treatment.

Nevertheless, symptoms can be controlled.

Symptom management options include:

Birth control tablets and loses weight

another androgen blocker, spironolactone

Metformin, a blood sugar-regulating medication, is frequently administered in addition to other fertility medications to aid in the induction of ovulation.

Note: If you become pregnant, you will need to stop taking some of these medications. Create a plan that works for you in collaboration with your physician.

Next actions

The most crucial fact regarding PCOS and pregnancy is the existence of serious difficulties. It is therefore more crucial than ever to take the necessary precautions to ensure a healthy pregnancy.

Consult your physician, adhere to a pregnancy-safe exercise and nutrition regimen, and take prescription drugs as prescribed. All of these treatment plans are advised for managing PCOS while pregnant.

Chapter 2:

Recognizing the Primary Cause of PCOS

The disorder known as PCOS, or polycystic ovarian syndrome, manifests as a variety of symptoms. It has many facets, and fresh information and variants on the topic are discovered every day. It can be difficult to fully comprehend PCOS given the abundance of information that is already available.

Gaining a deeper understanding of the underlying reasons for your PCOS might help you take steps towards managing and reversing the condition.

We shall examine the following four primary underlying causes of PCOS in this article:

- persistent inflammation
- Insulin sensitivity
- Adrenal and stress
- Androgen Overindulgence

1. **Chronic inflammation:** Previously believed to be a secondary effect of PCOS, new study indicates that a low-grade chronic inflammation may be a primary factor in the development of the disorder in a person.

One way to think of inflammation is as an immune system reaction. In order to protect the body against diseases and pathogens, the immune system often fights against them by releasing certain chemicals that cause an inflammatory reaction. For this reason, inflammation plays a crucial role in immunity. Throughout our lives, we oscillate between being pro- and anti-inflammatory. But inflammation is persistent in PCOS.

This is due to the fact that a person with PCOS is probably immune system weakened and has an excess of belly fat. This induces low-grade chronic inflammation by raising the body's level of alertness. This could be the primary cause of pain, exhaustion, stomach problems, and other symptoms, and it can go on for months or years.

Why does persistent inflammation occur?
Chronic inflammation results from an inflammatory response that persists despite you're no longer sick or injured. It's often seen in autoimmune conditions — such as lupus and rheumatoid arthritis — when the immune system mistakes your body's own tissues for a foreign threat. As opposed to acute while

chronic inflammation is a gradual process that might take months or years to resolve, (short-term) inflammation only lasts as long as your body needs to heal. Because it progresses more slowly and steadily rather than in a tidal wave, it is frequently referred to as low grade inflammation. The following factors may also contribute to chronic inflammation:

- Oxidative damage
- Fatness
- Emotional strain
- Elements of lifestyle
- Puffing

Can issues arise from PCOS and inflammation? PCOS-related low-grade inflammation raises the possibility of a number of health issues.

Infertility

Chronic inflammation can make it more difficult to get pregnant if you have PCOS. In particular, inflammation may interfere with your ovaries' ability to function normally.

Ovulation can be disrupted by PCOS, which reduces the likelihood that your ovaries will release a viable egg. Additionally, it may obstruct the process of implantation, which is when a fertilized embryo burrows into the uterine walls and starts to grow.

Diabetes type 2

Before the age of 40, type 2 diabetes strikes more than half of women with PCOS, according to the Centers for Disease Control and Prevention (CDC). This indicates that the prevalence of type 2 diabetes is significantly higher in PCOS patients than in non-PCOS patients.

According to a significant study, women with PCOS had a four times higher risk of type 2 diabetes than women without PCOS. Type 2 diabetes is influenced by insulin resistance, chronic inflammation, and excess weight.

Heart conditions

Individuals with PCOS are more vulnerable. Heart illness from a reliable source. Over time, inflammation-related oxidative stress can hurt your heart. Individuals with PCOS are also more likely to get high blood pressure and stroke.

Reducing inflammation through alterations in lifestyle

Reducing inflammation inside your body can assist in reducing the likelihood of PCOS issues.

PCOS anti-inflammatory diet

An anti-inflammatory diet is something that some people decide to do to control their PCOS symptoms and reduce their chance of consequences. Finding an anti-inflammatory diet that works for you may require some trial and error because each person's body reacts differently to different foods. However, some meals tend to reduce inflammation, but most meals tend to increase it.

Eating a diversified diet high in vitamins, minerals, and antioxidants is a good general rule of thumb. Rather than cutting out entire food groupings, concentrate on consuming things that will fuel your body. That being stated, you might want to stay away from the following foods that cause inflammation:

- Refined carbs found in cakes, donuts, pastries, and white bread, Cheese, milk, and other dairy items
- Sugar-filled drinks and snacks
- Finished meats
- Beverages
- Foods that have been preserved.

Exercise

Regular exercise can help people with PCOS reduce their risk of problems. Exercise can help you maintain a healthy weight, reduce inflammation, and enhance insulin resistance.

Frequent exercise also reduces the risk of heart disease and type 2 diabetes.

Studies indicate that the best outcomes for those with PCOS come from robust, intense exercise. Studies indicate that engaging in at least 120 minutes of intense exercise per week can lower your risk of PCOS issues. This can involve items like:

- Running
- Swimming
- Classes that use high-intensity interval training (HIIT)
- 360-degree Kickboxing

Other methods for reducing inflammation

Using holistic techniques, you could also be able to reduce inflammation in your body. Although some treatments lack scientific support, they might nevertheless enhance your general health and well-being.

Among these tactics are:

- Consuming dietary supplements that reduce inflammation, such as those containing ginger, spirulina, fish oil, and vitamin D
- Attempting acupuncture therapies
- Meditating regularly can help you manage stress and anxiety.
- Lowering the amount of chemicals, endocrine disruptors, air pollution, and other environmental pollutants that you are exposed to.

The conclusion

There is no distinct kind of PCOS other than inflammatory PCOS. Chronic inflammation is high in the majority of PCOS patients. PCOS and chronic inflammation are associated with several possible side effects, such as type 2 diabetes and obesity. Making lifestyle adjustments that lessen inflammation in your body may help you control the symptoms of PCOS and minimize the likelihood of problems.

2. Insulin Resistance:

Everyone must keep their blood sugar levels within the ideal range. The organ pancreas secretes insulin, which aids in controlling and storing glucose in the body. Generally speaking, the body's glucose should be able to respond to insulin; if it can't, the insulin has become less sensitive.

Insulin resistance is a state in which the body still secretes insulin but no longer has the sensitivity to use it properly. When this happens, the body tries to counteract by secreting more insulin, which results in hyperinsulinemia, or an excess of insulin in the blood. Elevated insulin can impede the ovaries' normal function, making PCOS more difficult to treat. Insulin resistance typically manifests as weight increase around the abdomen, skin tags, acanthosis, velvety dark patchy skin, difficulties decreasing weight, and cravings for sugar and carbohydrates.

Primary Factor in Insulin Resistance.

Research is still ongoing to determine the true reason why PCOS patients develop insulin resistance. Nonetheless, it has been discovered that the primary reason for the body's elevated insulin levels is insulin resistance brought on by PCOS.

Elevated insulin levels may stimulate the ovaries to generate more androgen hormones, potentially leading to symptoms such as irritability, inflammation, mood swings, and facial hair.

Moreover, insulin resistance associated with polycystic ovarian syndrome impairs cells' capacity to use insulin, resulting in elevated blood sugar levels and type 2 diabetes.

Indications of Resistance to Insulin PCR-based

Forty-five to seventy percent of women with PCOS exhibit symptoms of insulin resistance, including infertility, painful menstruation, and heavy bleeding. Because of an increase in testosterone production, elevated insulin levels exacerbate these symptoms. Weight gain around the waist and increased facial hair development are two more signs of insulin resistance PCOS. One of the most prevalent signs of PCOS is the presence of dark spots on the skin around the waist, neck, armpits, and groin area.

In addition, other indicators of PCOS insulin resistance, such as elevated insulin levels, contribute to chronic illnesses like diabetes, hypertension, obesity, and cardiac problems. Additionally, the illness could increase the desire for carbohydrates and sweets.

Symptoms of Insulin Resistance in PCOS

The signs of insulin resistance differ from woman to woman. These signs hardly ever noticed in small amounts. Among these signs and symptoms are:

- A craving for salty, sweet and carbohydrate meals.
- Tiredness.
- Darkening of the skin in the armpit, groin, and back of the neck.
- Frequent urge to take a shower.
- Thirst and hunger are increased.
- Tingling in the feet and hands.

Once you notice signs of PCOS insulin resistance, speak with your doctor about the next steps.

Diet for Insulin Resistance in PCOS

It becomes crucial to comprehend the fundamental core cause of PCOS to create an insulin-resistant diet. Everybody has a different diet depending on their lifestyle. For this reason, it's critical to have a solid understanding of the different nutrients we consume.

A patient's diet plan for PCOS insulin resistance must take heart-healthy fats, proteins, and the proper amount and kind of carbohydrates into consideration. The secret to the ideal diet is to combine these three nutrients in the right ratio. Here are some important things to keep in mind when creating a diet for women who exhibit insulin resistance symptoms associated with PCOS.

Select healthy carbohydrates like whole grains, which increase dietary fiber levels and aid in controlling blood sugar.

Reduce your carbohydrate intake to address the insulin resistance issue.

To lessen the amount of glucose your body is exposed to while fighting PCOS insulin resistance, incorporate the following foods into your meals.

- ¼ served with whole grains such as multigrain bread, brown rice, quinoa, or whole grain pasta.
- Produce Fruits
- A small amount of heart-healthy fats, including olive or nut oils
- Trimmed proteins.

By controlling the symptoms, women with PCOS insulin resistance can benefit from adhering to this diet.

3. Stress and Adrenals:

If you were held captive, how would you react at first? You will push back and resist, try to defend yourself as much as you can, and eventually come to a point where you will stop fighting and leave things up to fate. This same type of association exists between stress and PCOS. Stress is brought on by the hormone cortisol, which is released by the adrenal glands. Cortisol production is significantly higher in people with PCOS than in those without the condition.

It is a vicious cycle where stress is what sets off your PCOS and your PCOS in turn. This is due to the fact that elevated blood cortisol levels impact hormonal balance and function. It may alter your level of insulin resistance and initiate long-term, low-level inflammation.

Hormonal imbalance is the root cause of PCOS, and elevated blood cortisol levels impair normal hormone function. A direct correlation has been found between the low-grade chronic inflammation associated with PCOS and the rise in cortisol levels, which exacerbates insulin resistance. Therefore, adrenal stress is a double-edged blade that exacerbates an already difficult circumstance. A weakened immune system, anxiety, depression, fatigue in the morning, droop in the afternoon; and so on are signs that your adrenal glands are overworked.

Reasons behind Adrenal PCOS

Adrenal glands are located above the kidneys in the human body. In addition to producing adrenaline and norepinephrine, these glands primarily generate steroids, specifically glucocorticoids and mineralocorticoids. The majority of the hormones released by the adrenal glands are involved in the stress response, among other things.

When the body or mind is under stress, the pituitary releases ACTH, which instructs the adrenal glands to release DHEA and cortisol.

Describe DHEA.

The hormone DHEA is generated by each kidney's adrenal glands. It serves as a precursor for the production of other hormones, such as testosterone in males and estrogen in women.

Your natural DHEA levels are highest while you're a young adult. With aging, these levels decrease. To find out how well your adrenal glands are functioning and how much DHEA-S is in your blood, doctors run a DHEA-S test.

While excessive DHEA in males has no effect, in women, it can lead to symptoms like frank virilization, acne, hair loss or gain, irregular or missing periods, and fertility problems. High DHEA levels in younger children can cause an early onset of adrenarche or the activation of the adrenal gland.

How does DHEA relate to stress?

The human body often goes through a sequence of reactions when under stress in an attempt to manage the circumstances. The brain and hormones from the adrenal glands are two of the body's many components that are typically involved in this process. To specifically address stress in the body, the adrenal glands release DHEA and cortisol, the main stress hormone.

The body's regular processes may be impacted by extended activation of the stress response system and excessive exposure to stress hormones such as cortisol, DHEA, and others.

Signs of PCOS in the adrenals

When they first start menstruating in their teens or when they intend to get pregnant, most women start to notice signs of adrenal PCOS.

Typical PCOS symptoms and indicators include:

- Gaining weight
- Hair growth or loss
- Skin
- missing or irregular menstrual cycle

Adrenal Medications for PCOS

Adrenal PCOS is typically treated with lifestyle modifications. For example, studies have shown that reducing your body weight by up to 10% can help control your menstrual cycle and ease typical symptoms of PCOS. Eating a healthy, well-balanced diet makes this feasible.

Additionally, you can enhance your weight loss journey by working out three days a week. For best outcomes, adhere to the AHA/CDC physical activity guidelines.

Adults should perform 150–300 minutes of moderate aerobic exercise or 75–150 minutes of intense aerobic exercise per week, according to these recommendations for physical activity.

Depending on whether the lady wishes to become pregnant, there are also several efficient medicinal therapies available for adrenal PCOS. Typical medical interventions consist of:

1. Using contraceptive tablets

Using metformin to enhance hirsutism and insulin function.

Clomiphene to improve fertility in women attempting to conceive

Ovarian drilling is a medical technique that helps women resume normal ovulation

Strategies for stress management to control adrenal PCOS.

Restoring normal ovarian, insulin and menstrual function is essential for treating adrenal PCOS effectively. Healthily resolving stress can help with all of them. These could consist of the following:

2. Obtain restful slumber.

Your health is adversely affected by sleep loss. Research indicates that sleep deprivation may increase DHEA and cortisol levels. So, setting a goal of seven to eight hours of sleep per night is an easy yet effective intervention you may start doing immediately.

For uninterrupted sleep, you should keep electronics away from your sleeping space. Avoiding caffeine, cigarettes, and alcohol at least an hour before bed is also advised.

3. Regularly meditate.

Women with adrenal PCOS may find it helpful to meditate every day in addition to eating a healthy diet to control their stress levels. It not only relieves physical tension but also enhances the quality of your slumber by calming your mind and enabling you to concentrate on your dreams.

One of the most important parts of practicing meditation is learning the correct deep breathing techniques.

4. Work out

Exercise regimens that are mild and restorative can be highly helpful in reducing daily stress. Exercise—particularly endurance training—can also assist in regaining insulin sensitivity and healthy reproductive function.

5. Exercise self-care.

One of the best ways to relax and reduce stress is to take a few minutes for yourself. Everything that calms you down and enhances your mental health should be a part of a good self-care routine.

But this isn't limited to long baths and candles. Reading a book, going to a movie, spending time in nature, hanging out with friends and family, or even taking up a new activity are examples of further self-care practices.

4. **Androgen Overindulgence**:

Defining Androgens?

Androgens are vital hormones that support the following processes:

- Heart health Bone vigor
- Mass and tone of muscles
- Brain activity
- Libido, or the want to have sex
- Action and location of fat cells
- Growth of body and pubic hair

Androgen hormones are produced by the ovaries and fat cells that are allocated female at birth. They are also produced in the adrenal glands, which are in charge of releasing several hormones and are situated above the kidneys.

Unwanted hair growth is nothing new for those who have PCOS. There is male pattern hair growth and excessive hair loss in different body areas. The one responsible for

Androgens, or the male hormones released in excess in PCOS, are the cause of these abnormalities.

What Indices and Symptoms Point to an Androgen Overabundance?

Male-pattern baldness, abnormal hair growth, acne, and virilization—the process by which assigned females take on characteristics associated with assigned males—are among the indications and symptoms of hyperandrogenism.

Unexplained Hair Growth

Male-pattern hair development in females can indicate hyperandrogenism. Examples of this include hair on the chest, back, and face. This is known as hirsutism in medicine. About 5% to 10% of assigned females are affected by hirsutism.

One common symptom of PCOS is hirsutism. Some people, meanwhile, can have hirsutism without having PCOS. While rare, hirsutism can also develop in those suffering from illnesses involving the overproduction of male hormones or problems with the adrenal glands.

Some people may remove this kind of hair growth without realizing it could be an indication of a medical concern. Make sure you let your healthcare professional know if you're having this problem.

1. Skin

Mild acne in adults is not regarded as abnormal. On the other hand, moderate to severe acne may be a sign of elevated androgen levels, particularly if it is accompanied by other symptoms.

2. Absence of menstrual cycles

Amenorrhea, the cessation of the menstrual cycle, is a disorder caused by high levels of testosterone. There have been cases of amenorrhea in PCOS patients. Menstruation may also stop as a result of adrenal tumors.

3. Pattern Balding in Men

With aging, people may start to lose their hair. On the other hand, allocated females may have hyperandrogenism if they exhibit hair loss that resembles "male-pattern balding.

Male-pattern balding is characterized by hair loss around the top of the head or by the hairline, which causes the hairline to recede. This is not the same as female-pattern balding, in which the hairline itself stays the same but the hair on top of the head thins out.

4. Oily Skin: Androgens increase the skin's oil gland activity. Oily skin is the result of your oil glands releasing more sebum when they are more active.

Skin that has some sebum on it is more moisturized and protected. On the other hand, acne can result from pore blockages caused by excessive sebum production.

5. Sexualization

Virilization is the process by which assigned females acquire characteristics linked to assigned men. These alterations in assigned girls may be specifically caused by excess testosterone production.

Male-pattern hair growth, greasy skin, and irregular menstrual cycles can all be symptoms of low testosterone. While high levels can produce clitoris enlargement, deepening of the voice, and male muscle pattern, moderate levels can cause male-pattern baldness, loss of female fat distribution, and decreased breast size.

Normal Androgen Ranges

Total testosterone refers to the entire quantity of testosterone present in your blood. In allocated girls, levels should range from 6.0 to 86 nanograms per deciliter (ng/dl). Total testosterone may be slightly higher in PCOS.

Free testosterone: A little portion of total testosterone is this form of testosterone that is not bound to any proteins. In milliliters (pg/mL), free testosterone levels typically range from 0.7 to 3.6. PCOS patients may have higher levels of free testosterone.

Androstenedione: In assigned females, normal ranges are 0.7–3.1 ng/mL. Increased values could be a sign of PCOS.

DHEAS: A normal level for assigned girls in their 20s is often in the upper 300s. Individuals in their 30s might have 200s typical levels.

What Other Things Could Raise Your Androgen Levels?

PCOS affects most assigned females with hyperandrogenism. However, there are more potential reasons of hyperandrogenism that may result in PCOS-like symptoms:

A set of hereditary disorders known as congenital adrenal hyperplasia occur when the body lacks specific enzymes necessary for the synthesis of hormones. Together with other hormones, these disorders can have an effect on the adrenal glands and the body's capacity to produce androgens.

When the body produces too much cortisol, a stress hormone, either naturally or by prescription, Cushing's disease develops. Growths in the pituitary or adrenal glands, which assist in regulating hormones, might result in overproduction. High quantities of a hormone that aids in the manufacture of cortisol, which might raise androgens, may result from this growth.

Your ovaries may create too much testosterone if you have an ovarian tumor. Bloating, pelvic or belly pain, difficulty eating or feeling full quickly, and an overwhelming urge to urinate or Urinating frequently is one of the symptoms of ovarian cancer.

Hormone fluctuations can result from adrenal gland tumors. Elevated testosterone levels resulting from tumors secreting androgen can cause hair growth on the face and body, a receding hairline, irregular menstruation cycles, and a deepening of the female voice.

Which Health Problems Are Induced by Elevated Androgens?

Increased androgen levels in assigned girls can cause irregular periods, facial hair growth, and trouble getting pregnant. Some other risk factors that frequently coexist with PCOS are also brought on by these elevated levels.

Distribution of Fat

The location of fat storage in the body appears to be influenced by androgens. High testosterone-assigned females may begin to gain extra body fat around their abdomens. As a result, the body alters shape, with the belly bearing more weight.

Dietary factors can also influence hyperandrogenism. According to one study, worse diets are linked to increased rates of insulin resistance, obesity, and androgen excess. Individuals who ate a DASH or Mediterranean diet typically had lower levels of testosterone.

Resistance to Insulin

Admitted girls with extra androgens are at a higher risk of developing insulin resistance. When the body doesn't react to the hormone insulin as it should, it might lead to insulin resistance. Insulin aids in controlling blood sugar levels.

PCOS is also linked to insulin resistance. Not all PCOS patients, though, will become insulin resistant. Antiandrogen therapy has the potential to reverse insulin resistance in those who qualify.

Elevated blood sugar levels can be a result of insulin resistance. Significant harm can be caused by high blood sugar levels. There are high blood levels of insulin in people who are resistant to it. Type 2 diabetes and prediabetes can develop as a result of elevated blood insulin levels.

Cardio logical Issues

In assigned females, an elevated risk of cardiac issues is linked to unusually high levels of androgens.

Researchers are still working to understand the subtleties of how elevated androgen levels impact heart function. It appears that elevated androgen levels by themselves do not appear to raise the risk of cardiovascular issues. However, hyperandrogenism may raise your risk of heart attack, coronary heart disease, and cardiovascular disease when associated with irregular menstruation.

Obstacles during Pregnancy

It is well recognized that some persons with PCOS may become infertile. But many people with PCOS are nevertheless able to conceive. If conception does take place, there can be more dangers. Elevated testosterone levels can impact the ovaries and uterus, perhaps leading to premature birth, preeclampsia, and an inability of the embryo to adhere to the uterine wall. Additionally, it may make gestational diabetes more likely.

Everybody Has a Different Root Cause!

Various combinations of these underlying factors may be responsible for the symptoms that define your specific PCOS experience. Depending on the underlying cause or causes, several treatment strategies using diet, lifestyle, and specific supplements are used.

Furthermore, the majority of women's PCOS symptoms are caused by multiple underlying causes!

It is essential to engage with a professional who can assist you in identifying and treating YOUR root causes, as each person's root causes are unique and might occur in combination. When it comes to PCOS, there is no one size fits all solution!

Other Elements

Apart from these four, a person may be more susceptible to having PCOS due to additional dietary and environmental variables. Some of the environmental factors that contribute to PCOS include consuming large amounts of processed and canned foods, including inorganic foods in the diet, frequently using plastic containers, being around skin care products that contain parabens and phthalates, and being around pesticides. Creating a clean atmosphere and adopting healthy eating practices could be beneficial changes that someone can do to help manage their PCOS.

Uvi Health is a firm believer in addressing the underlying reasons of PCOS, getting to the core of the issue, and making changes. We've created a quiz to assist you in identifying the underlying reason for your PCOS. You'll be able to enhance your life quality and permanently alleviate your PCOS symptoms by doing this!

Chapter 3

PCOS Pregnancy and Ovulation

Polycystic ovarian syndrome, or PCOS, is a prevalent cause of female infertility and an ovulation.

It is also known as polycystic ovarian disease (PCOD) or PCO (polycystic ovaries).

Women experiencing infertility due to polycystic ovaries:

- Don't ovulate regularly
- Possess several tiny cystic structures in their ovaries, measuring between 2 and 9 mm in diameter.

How does ovulation normally occur?

A mature follicle, which is a cystic structure as well, develops throughout a typical menstrual cycle that includes ovulation. A developed follicle with a diameter of 18 to 28 mm is prepared for ovulation.

- If the lady is not pregnant, she should expect to have her period about 14 days after ovulation.
- The main distinction between ovaries that are polycystic and those that are normal is

that, while polycystic ovaries have a large number of tiny antral follicles containing eggs, these follicles do not mature and grow normally, which results in no ovulation.

- Women who have polycystic ovaries experience irregular menstrual cycles because they do not ovulate frequently.

What is the PCOS-related infertility rate?

With polycystic ovaries, the rate of infertility is extremely high. These women typically have trouble becoming pregnant, and they typically need treatment to increase their chances.

With polycystic ovarian syndrome, some women ovulate (produce a mature egg) on occasion, while others never do. We must ovulate for sperm to identify and fertilize a mature egg, which is necessary for conception.

Can women with PCOS become pregnant?

Fortunately, there is a high likelihood of becoming pregnant with polycystic ovarian syndrome while taking fertility medications. With fertility medication, the vast majority of women with polycystic ovarian syndrome will be able to conceive.

The main concern for young women with polycystic ovaries under 35 is not whether any medication would ever work, but rather which one will be effective.

Without knowing the specifics of each case, it is difficult to provide statistics regarding the likelihood of getting pregnant with PCOS.

Therapies for infertility and polycystic ovaries.

To conceive, women with polycystic ovarian syndrome typically require ovulation induction.

Details regarding options: Options for Treating PCOS Fertility and Their Success Rates.

Options for treating PCOS fertility include:

1. For PCOS, Clomid
2. For PCOS, use Femara (Letrozole).
3. PCOS with Metformin
4. PCOS Injectable Gonadotropins
5. PCOS In Vitro Fertilization (IVF)

How to Determine Whether PCOS Is Causing Regular Ovulation

Many women who struggle with conception would likely concur that determining the cause is essential to putting an end to their frustration.

Your menstrual cycle and capacity to ovulate can be affected by polycystic ovarian syndrome (PCOS), which can make it difficult to conceive. But don't worry; there are methods for determining if you are ovulating.

Ovulation and PCOS

The brain secretes a specific hormone that triggers the menstrual cycle. In the end, this results in the ovary's egg follicle starting to grow.

This mechanism involves two primary hormones. Follicle-stimulating hormone (FSH) is the first; it promotes an egg's maturation. Luteinizing hormone (LH) is the second, and it is responsible for inducing ovulation, or the release of the egg.

The eggs of PCOS-affected women don't always develop or come out of the ovary to be fertilized. Instead, as tiny, immature follicles, they gather on the ovaries. They are incorrectly referred to as cysts.

Excess androgen production is common in PCOS-affected women. Ovulation and a woman's menstrual cycle may be impacted as a result.

She might have irregular or longer-than-normal cycles. They might also not happen at all. In a certain cycle, she might or might not ovulate.

It is challenging to determine whether or not ovulation is taking place during these erratic cycles.

This will impact the fertility of a woman. This is also a prevalent issue in the US. According to data from the Centers for Disease Control and Prevention, about 19% of women between the ages of 15 and 49 are infertile. (Being infertile is defined as not getting pregnant after a year of trying.)

In the same age range, about 26% of women had difficulties becoming pregnant or bringing a child to term. This condition is known as "impaired fecundity."

Indication of ovulation

One indication of ovulation is regular menstruation. To increase your chances of becoming pregnant, you can determine when and if you are ovulating by:

- Buying a kit for predicting ovulation.
- It can identify increased amounts of LH, which peaks just before ovulation. The levels of LH in women with PCOS are often high. For this reason, a kit might not be as trustworthy for them as it is for other ladies.
- Determining your body's baseline temperature
- Taking your temperature while at rest is another method to find out if you're ovulating. A progesterone surge causes your basal body temperature to rise by around one degree between one and three days

following ovulation. Use a digital thermometer as soon as you wake up and before you get out of bed to ensure reliable readings.

Examining your cervical secretions:

The cervical mucus of a woman varies during her monthly menstrual cycle. She will have dry cervical mucus at the beginning of her period. Ovulation may be on the verge when cervical mucus is moist or has the consistency of raw egg whites.

Finding the cervical position yourself:

Your cervix also changes as your menstrual cycle advances each month. Reach within your vagina to feel your cervix. If you can feel your cervix quite readily, you are generally not near to ovulating.

Take a look at these tactics each month to learn more about your body. They might make it more likely for you to become pregnant.

If you're trying to get pregnant, using one or more of these methods can help you figure out when to schedule sex appropriately. The "fertile window" usually lasts for approximately one day following ovulation and starts five days prior. Ovulation timing might vary, so you might want to start trying a week or so before you think you'll ovulate and keep trying for a few days after that.

Try these strategies every month and get to know your body. They might make it more likely for you to become pregnant.

In Case you're Unsure

See a doctor and have an assessment if you don't receive any obvious signs that you're ovulating. You might require assistance controlling your menstrual cycles or conceiving.

A reproductive endocrinologist or fertility expert will often do an ultrasound, obtain a thorough medical history, and perform a complete hormone workup. You can use these steps to find out when and if you are ovulating.

5 Strategies to Increase Fertility and Conceive With PCOS

A common worry among women with polycystic ovarian syndrome (PCOS) is becoming pregnant. One of the most prevalent disorders among infertile women is PCOS. The androgen hormones, which are male hormones, are more prevalent in women with this illness. The ovulation process may be hampered by this hormone imbalance. PCOS can make getting pregnant more difficult, but there are options for women to increase their fertility.

1. **Medications can be required.**

A good ovulation process may be hampered by high testosterone levels. A woman cannot become pregnant if a healthy egg is not produced during ovulation. Many women with PCOS require ovulation-inducing medicines to conceive. These drugs may facilitate a woman's ovulation and subsequent conception. Women can identify the ideal medicine type and dosage by consulting with a healthcare professional or fertility specialist.

2. **Determine Your Fit Weight**

Many women discover that even a 10% weight loss might enhance their ovulation and hormone levels. A woman's overall fertility, insulin resistance, and menstrual cycle can all be improved with even a small body weight loss of 5%. According to one study, women who exercised daily were 5% less likely to become infertile than those who did not. On the other hand, excessive exercise might cause the body to become more inflammatory, which is bad for fertility. Try to work out three days a week at a moderate level for the best effects.

3. **Lessen Stress**

It might be difficult to manage stress when facing infertility. However, chronic stress can negatively affect hormones and fertility. Excessive stress raises cortisol levels, which might cause an increase in insulin. For those who have trouble managing their stress, talk therapy, meditation, exercise, and spending time with loved ones can all be beneficial.

4. Use Aided Reproduction Techniques

Women may benefit from assisted reproductive technologies (ART), such as in vitro fertilization (IVF), if ovulation drugs are ineffective in increasing fertility. According to studies, the success rates for IVF treatments among women with PCOS are comparable to those of women without the illness. To increase fertility, doctors typically start with medication and lifestyle modifications. If these methods are unsuccessful, they may then suggest ART.

5. Medical Choices

Women with PCOS can enhance their fertility through surgical procedures if other treatment choices prove ineffective. Ovarian drilling is one type of surgery used to induce ovulation. Research has shown that up to 50% of women who have ovarian drilling can become pregnant within the first year following the procedure, even though it is not usually required.

Avoid Loss of Hope

In the US, approximately 10% of women suffer from PCOS. Even though the illness may make pregnancy more difficult, women shouldn't give up hope because having a child is still possible. If a woman with PCOS wishes to get pregnant, she should speak with a doctor about her diagnosis and available treatments.

Chapter 4:

How to Reverse PCOS and What You Should Know

Indeed, PCOS can be reversed without the need for medication. This is how

If you're taking pills for PCOS and its bothering you, it's time to reverse it naturally with a few lifestyle adjustments.

PCOS affects a large number of women and young girls nowadays. Additionally, food and lifestyle-related issues contribute to PCOS, as they do to most diseases. For this reason, making dietary and lifestyle modifications should be the first line of successful treatment rather than taking birth control pills!

Before I started exploring the world of healing and nutrition, I struggled with PCOS for a long time. That's how I was able to heal my illness naturally and without medicine. Because they directly affect our biology, dietary changes can have a significant influence on our health.

If you have endometriosis, fibroids, PCOS, or any other hormonal condition, there are natural remedies you can try. Think of this as the definitive PCOS diet guide:

1. Eat fewer foods high in glucose.

Your body's resistance to insulin exacerbates hormonal abnormalities, which in turn lead to PCOS. To ensure that your body receives adequate nourishment and fewer glucose spikes, include a variety of vegetables in your meals every day and consume foods with a low glycemic index, such as whole grains. Hormone-balancing foods include broccoli, cabbage, beans, lentils, mustard leaves, seeds, and more.

2. Add ghee to your meals.

I've never understood why people are afraid to eat ghee, considering it's been a staple of the Indian diet for so long! Ghee is excellent for lubricating your joints and regulating your hormones. It's also very good for the wellness of your brain. But be sure the ghee you eat is hormone- and antibiotic-free, and that it is derived from raw milk. Avoid purchasing low-cost factory-made copies.

3. Consume less milk.

Many people continue to consume milk and milk products despite having poor digestion. It's advisable to stay away from milk if your digestion isn't the best so that it doesn't affect your body.

4. Consume fewer fruits

Natural sugar content is very high in most fruits. If you already have insulin resistance, you should limit the amount of fruit you eat. Reduce them as much as you can until your body regains insulin sensitivity, but don't eliminate them.

5. Maintain a restricted eating window

It is crucial to fast for a few hours to allow your digestive system to rest and to make your body more sensitive to insulin. Several hours of fasting each day is an excellent method to achieve this.

6. Make your life more active

While most health conditions can be resolved with dietary modifications, improving your health is guaranteed when you combine a healthy diet with regular exercise. While excessive exercise is not necessary, moving in some capacity each day is!

7. Sun exposure

We take this for granted, and the majority of people I know never see the light either because of the layout of their homes, a lack of room, or just the fact that they stay indoors all the time. In addition to being essential for the synthesis of vitamin D, solar energy is also necessary for a healthy circadian rhythm. Spend at least thirty minutes each day in the sun.

Chronic illness cannot be cured by a miraculous drug. Over time, small daily adjustments add up to a great deal, and your body begins reacting to these adjustments almost instantly!

Six Steps to a Natural Reversal of PCOS

1. Have a hormone test performed

It's essential to get a full hormone test performed by your physician to determine the specific type of PCOS you have and which hormones require balancing. Some women may be estrogen dominant (meaning their progesterone levels are too low and estrogen levels are too high), which results in long menstrual cycles, heavy cramps, severe PMS symptoms, and infertility. Other women may have excess androgens (male hormones), which can cause acne, weight gain around the midsection, facial hair growth, and missed periods.

Make sure your physician performs a full panel, including measurements of estrogen, progesterone, testosterone, AMHA, DHEA, and maybe even your thyroid and insulin, since women with PCOS frequently have insulin resistance and hypothyroidism. (In addition, you can use this free test to determine whether you have PCOS while you wait to visit your doctor.)

2. Consume a diet low in inflammation

It's very astonishing how our nutrition affects our hormones. I minimized my consumption of gluten, dairy, inflammatory oils, sugar, and processed foods by adhering to an anti-inflammatory diet.

Rather, I piled my plate high with entire grains, vegetables, lean protein, healthy fats, and organic, high-fiber fruits. In addition, I consumed a lot of foods high in hormone-healing ingredients, such as collagen, apple cider vinegar, bone broth, cinnamon, spearmint tea, and nourishing teas.

3. Consume vitamins that balance hormones.

My supplement regimen is much simpler now, but it was crucial to feed my body a diverse range of vitamins, minerals, and other nutrients during the early phases of my recovery. I had doubts about the effectiveness of supplements, but I can honestly state that they played a major role in my recovery. Regardless of how healthful your diet is, there are certain minerals that our bodies just cannot absorb from food alone (like vitamin D!).

To be honest, finding the right supplement regimen takes some trial and error, but some of the hormone-balancing pills that I used to correct my PCOS were Maca, vitex, DIM, evening primrose oil, inositol, and magnesium.

4. Work out wisely

Did you know that running or exercising for longer than 60 minutes a day can cause your adrenal glands to burn out? And that having too much cortisol, the stress hormone, can throw off the balance of your other hormones?

That's why I changed from doing lengthy, tough workouts several times a week to doing shorter, daily workouts (15–30 minutes). In addition, I gave up running in favor of long, leisurely walks and healing yoga sessions. Self-care practices like massages, Epsom salt baths, meditation, and reading (especially outside for 15 minutes each day to increase vitamin D levels) are some other ways to nourish your adrenals. Reducing alcohol and caffeine consumption is also beneficial.

5. Get rid of harmful goods that mess with hormones

What we put on our bodies is just as vital as what we put inside of them. Sadly, the majority of store-bought items also include a concoction of dangerous chemicals that have been linked to hormone imbalances (including infertility), cancer, allergies, asthma, and neurotoxicity. Since many of these toxins in the body mimic estrogen, eliminating these products was very crucial for my

PCOS because they exacerbated estrogen dominance and hormonal imbalances.

Toxic skincare, makeup, personal hygiene, and cleaning supplies purchased from stores should be thrown away. Replace them with safe, natural alternatives.

I also began manufacturing a lot of my own cleaning and a skincare product, which is a very easy, very affordable way to ensure that the stuff you use won't interfere with your hormones.

6. Sync your blood sugar

Another problem that many women with PCOS have is insulin resistance. Essentially, you have a much higher chance of getting type 2 diabetes if your blood sugar (fasting glucose and insulin) levels are too high. I eliminated sugar and processed carbohydrates in favor of protein, fiber, and healthy fats to fight this.

I also reduced my fasting insulin levels by eating at regular intervals, particularly first thing in the morning. My blood sugar balanced so quickly with this method that I was almost shocked.

Final Reflections

And that's it, my friend. There are six natural strategies to reverse PCOS. Please take note that my suggestions do not replace the counsel of a licensed medical expert. Instead, I strongly advise you to choose a holistic physician you can trust who can handle your particular difficulties and guide you through the natural PCOS healing process.

It's important to remember that PCOS has no known "cure." I'll always possess it. I can handle it. I can effectively put the chronic illnesses that come with the hormone issue into reverse and put my symptoms into "remission." However, PCOS can always flare up again if I don't take proper care of my body, and I will have to live with this fact for the rest of my life.

However, I also know that if I follow these six steps again during a flare-up, my hormones will return to normal and my symptoms will go away in a matter of weeks.

Fruit Consumption to Reverse PCOS

Do Fruits Work Well For **PCOS**?

Fruits are wonderful! Fruit is naturally sweet and packed with health benefits. They therefore work wonders in assisting you in obtaining your recommended daily intake of vitamins, minerals, and antioxidants. They also satisfy your need for sweet treats!

The high fiber content of most fruits helps to prolong feelings of fullness by delaying the digestion of sugar. Another naturally occurring sugar that can be found in fruits is fructose. Sucrose is not as good as fructose as sugar.

Still, keep in mind that it is sugar, so pay attention to how much you eat and how you portion out your fruit. One effective strategy to reduce the rate at which sugar enters your bloodstream is to consume your fruit with nuts or your preferred protein. Research indicates that substituting fruit for your regular snacks will help reduce obesity, insulin resistance, and elevated blood sugar levels.

I used to have a continual sugar addiction, so I would always eat fruit as a snack. I was unaware that the fruit was increasing my appetite because it also contained sugar. As a registered dietitian, I now understand that if I matched

My blood sugar would have stabilized if I had paired my fruit with nuts, seeds, or my preferred protein, which would have greatly decreased my cravings.

Not all fruits are created equal, even if including fruits in your PCOS diet plan is an excellent idea.

The body will benefit from some of them more than others. Depending on the fruit, you'll want to choose ones with a low glycemic index (GI) and consume them with the skin on. That way, you'll always get more fiber and benefits!

I'll list 12 fruits below that may aid in weight loss, inflammation reduction, insulin level lowering, and other health benefits! Listed below are: Peaches, pears, watermelons, apples, cucumbers, mangoes, kiwis, bananas, oranges, and lemons can all be eaten with their skins on.

Fruits Friendly for PCOS

Apples

One of the best fruits for PCOS is apples! You can obtain the most health advantages without compromising flavor by eating them with the skin on. It's not a chore. In addition to being high in flavonoids, antioxidants, and vitamin C, apples aid indigestion.

These nutrients can lower inflammation, boost fertility, and control the menstrual cycle. Additionally, studies have demonstrated that apples can support hormone balance! I enjoy eating my apple with cocoa nibs and almond butter to help reduce the amount of sugar that enters my bloodstream.

Pears. Pears are Packed with potassium, iron, and vitamin C, pears also have a high fiber content. They're another fruit you can eat with the skin on, and they taste really good. Iron and vitamin C both aid in managing the menstrual cycle and exhaustion, respectively. Furthermore, fiber has been demonstrated to help control estrogen levels, reduce blood sugar, and remove toxins from the liver.

Orange-colored

Compared to several other fruits on this list, oranges have a lower fiber-to-sugar ratio, but if you eat the peel, you'll get an increased amount of fiber. (I enjoy putting them in smoothies.) Even so, a tiny peel-free orange won't harm you because they're a great source of vitamin C!

Kinki

Small as they are, kiwis have several health benefits for PCOS-affected women. According to studies, kiwis can protect our eyes, regulate digestion, control period discomfort, reduce inflammation, drop blood sugar, and even help with mood disorders.

All of these beneficial effects are possible because of the vitamin C, vitamin E, copper, vitamin K, magnesium, and potassium content of this potent fruit—which you should eat with the skin on!

Pecans

Eat your peaches with the skin on; you know the drill. Like the other fruits on this list, these stone fruits offer many of the same advantages. They do, however, include a few extra nutrients that may aid with hair loss, depression, cyst formation, inflammation, and insulin resistance. For an extra protein boost in the summer, I enjoy pairing peaches with prosciutto.

Berries

Who is not a grape lover? Antioxidants, fiber, foliate, potassium, calcium, magnesium, vitamin K, vitamin B, and vitamin C are all abundant in grapes. These little, bite-sized super foods can lower androgen levels in your body and improve ovarian health, which will help you create a more favorable environment for conception and pregnancy!

In addition, they may help regulate blood sugar and hormones, according to research. With so many health advantages and a very high GI score, grapes are a fantastic addition to any PCOS diet.

Sweet cherries: Due to their high potassium, fiber, and antioxidant content, cherries are another food that is good for PCOS. Your adrenal system will receive incredible support from this combo! Cherries have the potential to improve PCOS symptoms by lowering blood pressure, menstrual cycle regulation, and male hormone levels.

Grapes

Studies suggest that vitamin C may be necessary for a healthy menstrual cycle in women with PCOS. Additionally, vitamin C shields your body from free radicals, which may raise your risk of heart disease. The best thing, though? Vitamin C is abundant in grapefruit! Making it an extremely healthful option for PCOS sufferers.

Strawberry

Another delicious fruit that is beneficial for PCOS sufferers in terms of vitamins and nutrients is this one. Strawberries are high in potassium, folic acid, fiber, and vitamin C. When taken together, these minerals and vitamins can help increase good cholesterol and decrease blood pressure.

Cantaloupe: Be mindful of your portion sizes when eating melons, as they have a somewhat lower GI score than other fruits on this list. However, cantaloupe is often a delicious and healthful snack for people with PCOS! It contains fiber, magnesium, iron, vitamin B, and vitamin C. This suggests that cantaloupe may aid in hormone balance and fatigue reduction. Delicious and nutritious!

Papaya. Papayas are a tropical fruit that can be difficult to find depending on where you live, but if you do, they make a delicious snack. Because they contain more sugar, be mindful of how much you eat. There are tons of vitamins C, A, B, E, and K in every papaya! This combination of nutrients can assist you in controlling your menstrual cycle and mood.

Magnesium

Pomegranates are the final fruit on our list. Although you should only eat this fruit in moderation, it does include antioxidants, folate, potassium, magnesium, and calcium to assist your body stay strong and help you manage the

Symptoms of PCOS.

This is a list of indicators indicating PCOS is being reversed.

1. Your menstrual cycle will begin to regularize; 2. Your skin will clear up and the dark spots will start to fade;

3. Your acne will drastically transform;

4. You'll begin to lose weight;

5. You'll notice that the growth of unsightly facial hair has stopped;

6. You'll feel a lot more energized;

7. Your sleep will improve; and

8. You'll experience a reduction in tension. Anxiety and that's the way it's done! Are you prepared to stop the PCOS symptoms now?

Chapter 5:

What connection exists between insulin and PCOS?

Describe PCOS.

Reproductive hormone imbalances are the endocrine cause of PCOS. Almost 10% of women who are of reproductive age have PCOS. Although there isn't a particular test to identify PCOS, sufferers usually exhibit two or more of the following symptoms:

- Ovulation irregular or absent
- Lab tests reveal hyperandrogenism or high amounts of androgen.
- A large number of ovarian follicles

Every month, healthy ovaries release eggs. Ovarian issues, such as those associated with PCOS, might affect menstruation regularly and fertility. The primary cause of ovulatory infertility in women is PCOS.

Period irregularities could indicate irregular ovulation. Ultrasonography can identify physical abnormalities, such as an overabundance of ovarian follicles (follicles that are commonly referred to as cysts in PCOS).

An excess of androgens is known as hyperandrogenism. These are reproductive hormones, such as testosterone, which might interfere with ovulation and hinder the release of eggs from your body. Other symptoms that hyperandrogenism may be linked to include:

- Excessive facial and body hair growth, or hirsutism
- Alopecia (hair loss)
- Acne

There appear to be certain factors that raise the risk of developing PCOS, even though its causes are not entirely understood. You might have a higher chance of developing PCOS if you have a family history. The development of PCOS may also be influenced by lifestyle variables such as nutrition, exposure to pollutants in the environment, and inactivity.

PCOS and other metabolic disorders are closely associated. The metabolic syndrome's elements, such as obesity, insulin resistance, high blood pressure, and cholesterol, can also be present in PCOS patients.

What Is It Insulin Resistance? The pancreas Insulin Resistance secretes the hormone insulin, which aids in controlling blood glucose levels. Your blood glucose level increases after eating and insulin is released to transfer blood glucose into the cells. Glucose is the energy source that cells use to power bodily processes.

When your body produces enough insulin but is unable to use it efficiently, it might lead to insulin resistance. Blood glucose levels may therefore be greater than usual. In response, the body produces more insulin (hyperinsulinemia). Type 2 diabetes may occur if the pancreas is unable to produce enough insulin.

A new estimate puts the prevalence of insulin resistance in PCOS patients between 44% to 70%.

Data show that elevated fat cells, decreased serum adiponectin, and central abdominal weight are the best markers of insulin resistance in women with PCOS

Therefore, having extra weight around your abdomen may make you more vulnerable. The protein hormone adiponectin is generated by adipose tissue and plays a role in controlling blood sugar levels and insulin sensitivity.

Insulin Resistance Symptoms in PCOS-Affected Women

Even though insulin resistance may exist without any symptoms, there are occasionally warning indicators, such as:

Acanthosis nigricans: Thickening and darkening of the skin, usually in the folds around the groin, armpits, and neck.

Hunger: Excessive hunger may be a symptom of elevated insulin levels.

Gaining weight and having trouble reducing it: Insulin facilitates the body's storage of glucose for use as fuel in the muscles and liver. Excess glucose is stored as fat, which can make it difficult to lose weight and cause weight gain.

Screening for Insulin Resistance in PCOS-Affected Women

A lab test is not necessarily the best technique to diagnose insulin resistance. Because insulin resistance lab testing is intrusive and complex, it is often used in research settings. To find out if your body has high glucose levels, which could indicate that your body is having trouble processing blood sugar, there are tests available. They consist of:

Plasma glucose fasting: A lab draw is used to assess plasma glucose fasting (FPG) during fasting (typically in the morning before eating). FPG should not exceed 100 mg/dL. FPG is regarded as prediabetes, which is a risk factor for type 2 diabetes, if it is between 100 and 125 mg/dL. If

FPG is 126 mg/dL or higher, diabetes may be diagnosed.

A1C test: The A1C test, also called glycated hemoglobin or HbA1c, determines your average blood glucose level over the previous two to three months. A lab draw is used to assess the A1C to detect diabetes or prediabetes. A1C values in the range of 5.7% to 6.4% indicate prediabetes. If it's 6.5% or higher, a diabetes diagnosis might be made.

Oral glucose tolerance test (OGTT): This test measures the body's response to glucose and can be done in a lab or doctor's office. Two blood draws are made: one during the fast and the second two hours after consuming a glucose combination. An assessment of prediabetes is made if the values fall between 140 and 199 mg/dL. 200 mg/dL or higher is the threshold for the diagnosis of diabetes.

Insulin resistance may also be indicated by elevated fasting and/or two-hour insulin levels (reference values will vary slightly by laboratory).

The Homeostatic Model Assessment for Insulin Resistance, or HOMA-IR, is computed using insulin and fasting glucose levels. Insulin resistance is generally indicated by readings greater than 2, however, population-specific reference ranges may differ.

How Insulin Resistance Affects PCOS through Diet

In PCOS, diet can affect insulin resistance. During digestion, carbohydrates in food are converted to glucose. After the glucose enters the bloodstream, insulin transports it into the cell.

The need for insulin increases with the amount of carbohydrates consumed. Carbohydrate-containing foods include starchy vegetables, rice, pasta, cereal, oats, bread, fruit, and tortillas.

Opting for higher-fiber complex carbs and whole grains may be a better way to address insulin resistance. Foods high in fiber usually have a lower glycemic index (GI). Foods are ranked on the glycemic index based on how they affect blood glucose levels. Selecting low-GI foods instead of high-GI ones could help reduce insulin resistance.

Medications for PCOS Resistance to Insulin

PCOS can be treated even though it cannot be cured. Diabetes can be avoided and PCOS symptoms can be improved by treating insulin resistance.

Dietary changes and physical activity can improve insulin sensitivity, says Hieronymus. A healthy lifestyle can do this.

PCOS treatment entails:

Metformin: Your doctor may recommend metformin to assist in increasing your body's sensitivity to insulin, which helps lower testosterone levels and improve blood glucose levels. Ovulation regulation may also be aided by treating hyperandrogenism.

Myo-inositol supplementation: Nuts, fruits, grains, beans, and corn all contain isothiols. According to research, using a combination of myo- and D-chiro-inositol supplements may help PCOS patients regain ovulation, reduce their insulin levels, and improve their insulin resistance.

Diet: Research has indicated that a few dietary strategies can enhance insulin resistance. For those with PCOS, diets like the Mediterranean diet and the Dietary Approaches to Stop Hypertension (DASH) diet that emphasizes eating more fruits, vegetables, and healthy fats may offer a variety of health advantages.

Exercise: Exercise may help improve insulin resistance and reduce cardiovascular risk in PCOS patients. In addition, it might enhance mood and mental clarity, lower the chance of illness, increase stamina, and assist in managing current medical issues.

Weight loss: Reducing your body weight by merely 5% to 10% may help with insulin resistance and other symptoms associated with PCOS.

Hormonal birth control: If you have PCOS symptoms like acne and excessive hair growth, your doctor may prescribe birth control to help control your monthly cycle. It won't, however, have an impact on insulin resistance.

Insulin: In cases with more severe insulin resistance, this medication may be recommended.

The connection between insulin resistance and PCOS

Principal information to be aware of:

Most patients with polycystic ovarian syndrome (PCOS) have elevated insulin levels or insulin resistance.

High insulin has a physiological basis as well as being a sign of PCOS.

Insulin resistance testing can be useful in excluding other illnesses that are frequently misdiagnosed as PCOS.

Although the term "PCOS" implies that the condition is only related to the ovaries, it is not. Although PCOS affects the ovaries and the process of ovulation, it is a metabolic and endocrine illness that affects the entire body and is directly related to insulin resistance.

Insulin resistance: what is it?

Normal circumstances cause the hormone insulin to temporarily increase after eating. It encourages the muscles and liver to absorb blood sugar and transform it into energy. This consequently results in a drop in insulin and blood sugar. On a fasting blood test, insulin and sugar are both normal in those with normal insulin sensitivity.

Blood sugar may be normal in those with insulin resistance, but insulin is elevated. How come? Because to get its message across, the pancreas must produce an increasing amount of insulin. Excessive insulin leads to weight gain and inflammation. Heart disease and Type 2 diabetes might potentially result from it. Another physiological factor that underlies PCOS is an excess of insulin.

The connection between PCOS and insulin resistance

A crucial component of PCOS in both fat and lean individuals is insulin resistance. It affects 30–75% of those with lean PCOS and 70–95% of those with obese PCOS.

Excess insulin is a primary cause of PCOS as well as one of its symptoms. Excessive testosterone production from the ovaries and impaired ovulation can result from high insulin.

According to one study, within the past ten years, there has been a correlation between the prevalence of PCOS and a rise in obesity and weight gain. A "galloping increase of PCOS in parallel with the rising prevalence of type 2 diabetes" was reported in a different study.

Assessing insulin intolerance

I think it crucial to validate insulin resistance using a blood test, such as a 2-hour insulin glucose challenge test, HOMA-IR index, or fasting insulin, as a clinician who recommends diet and natural therapy for PCOS.

I can detect PCOS in individuals who do not have an insulin issue by testing for insulin resistance. Examples of these patients include the small group with adrenal PCOS and the very large group with hypothalamic amenorrhea who have been mistakenly labeled as having "lean PCOS."

Traditional therapy for PCOS and insulin resistance

Losing weight, engaging in aerobic activity, and taking the diabetes medication metformin—which increases insulin sensitivity—are the standard therapy recommendations for the insulin resistance component of PCOS. Further research is necessary to determine the effectiveness of resistance training.

The only officially suggested treatment for PCOS is oral contraceptives, yet these may interfere with the insulin resistance and sugar management that cause PCOS (13). It has been said that there is a "modern medical quandary" involving PCOS, insulin resistance, and oral contraceptive pill use that requires more investigation.

Fructose's part in insulin resistance

Reducing sugar is, in my opinion, the most successful dietary strategy for my PCOS patients.

Fructose in and of itself is safe; excessive amounts can be harmful. For instance, low-dose sugar from fruit improves insulin sensitivity and health rather than causing insulin resistance. Fruit juice, soft drinks, and pastries that contain high doses of fructose have a completely different impact. One researcher said, "There is a fundamental physiological difference in the way the body processes larger and smaller amounts of sugar." When fructose is consumed in excess, it can overpower the small intestine's natural processing mechanisms and make its way to the liver, where it can cause inflammation and reduce insulin sensitivity. This requires further investigation.

Nutritional supplements to treat PCOS and insulin resistance.

Myo- and di-chiro inositol are two forms of inositol that can be taken as a dietary supplement. One intracellular messenger implicated in insulin signaling is isothiol. According to a 2018 meta-analysis of 10 randomized trials, inositol appears to regulate menstrual cycles, promote ovulation, and trigger metabolic changes in patients with polycystic ovarian syndrome in addition to dramatically improving markers of insulin resistance. The majority of the randomized trials employed doses between 1.2 and 4 grams daily.

My second favorite supplement for insulin resistance is magnesium since it addresses the common subclinical magnesium shortage that some experts believe may be a factor in heart disease and insulin resistance. At least one-third of people, if not more, suffer from magnesium insufficiency, which is difficult to identify by a blood test.

One small study found that co-supplementing magnesium, zinc, calcium, and vitamin D improved the insulin metabolism of PCOS patients. A recent meta-analysis concluded that magnesium supplementation helps treat insulin resistance in adults with magnesium insufficiency.

Why does insulin resistance frequently coexist with PCOS?

Though PCOS exacerbates insulin resistance, it is hypothesized that insulin resistance precedes PCOS.

Regarding the mechanism by which insulin resistance leads to PCOS, several experts believe that persistently elevated insulin levels in the bloodstream stimulate the ovaries to produce more androgens. Insulin is a hormone, and hormone imbalances can throw other hormones into disarray.

It's crucial to note that insulin resistance is not the only route to PCOS development; the disease can also arise from other causes.

Let's return to that cycle now. The additional male hormones that follow PCOS cause fat to build around the abdomen. As you may have observed, women are more inclined to accumulate fat at the hips than males are to do the same around the abdomen. The body reacts differently to male and female hormones, which is why.

As I've previously mentioned, fat cells surrounding the abdominal organs are known to produce more cytokines, which are proteins. These cytokines cause insulin receptors to malfunction normally and become more resistant to insulin.

To put it another way, elevated insulin levels exacerbate PCOS. PCOS-related increases in androgens can result in weight gain around the abdomen, which exacerbates insulin resistance.

Chapter 6

Hormones and PCOS

Women of reproductive age are affected by the complicated endocrine condition known as polycystic ovarian syndrome, or PCOS. Hormonal imbalances are its defining feature, and they have a big impact on metabolism, reproductive health, and general well-being. The roles of estrogen, progesterone, and androgens in PCOS will be thoroughly examined in this article, along with their effects on the onset and course of the illness.

PCOS Hormonal Imbalance.

Estrogen Imbalance: An essential female hormone, estrogen, is responsible for controlling the menstrual cycle and preserving reproductive health. Estrogen levels frequently rise in PCOS for a variety of reasons. The ovaries' excessive synthesis of estrogen is one of the main causes of increased estrogen in PCOS. Elevated estrogen levels are also a result of poor metabolism and disturbed hormonal feedback mechanisms. An ovulation, or the absence of ovulation, and irregular menstrual periods can result from a persistent increase in estrogen. Moreover, endometrial hyperplasia and cancer risk are correlated with consistently elevated estrogen levels in PCOS.

Progesterone deficiency: Referred to as the "pregnancy hormone," progesterone plays a crucial role in assisting conception and readying the uterus for implantation. Progesterone deficiencies are frequently associated with PCOS because of erratic or nonexistent ovulation. This results in insufficient progesterone production during the second half of the menstrual cycle, a condition known as luteal phase deficit. In women with PCOS, progesterone shortage increases the chance of miscarriage, makes conceiving harder, and causes irregular menstruation. To improve reproductive results and restore hormonal balance, it is imperative to address this insufficiency.

The function of androgens: This class of hormones, which includes testosterone, is normally found in both males and females. However, women with PCOS frequently have higher testosterone and androgen levels. The body's delicate hormonal balance is upset by the higher androgens, which also contributes to the development of symptoms associated with hormonal imbalance in female PCOS patients. An overabundance of androgens can interfere with follicular growth, which can result in irregular menstrual cycles and the creation of ovarian cysts. High androgen levels can also cause acne, male-pattern hair loss, hirsutism, or excessive hair growth. Controlling androgen levels is essential for reducing symptoms of hormonal imbalance in females and enhancing the general health of PCOS-affected women.

It is essential to comprehend how these hormones interact to properly manage PCOS. A variety of hormonal imbalance therapy strategies, such as medication, hormonal treatments, and lifestyle changes, can be used to treat hormonal imbalances in PCOS. Adjusting one's lifestyle to a healthy weight, getting frequent exercise, and eating balanced food can all help to better regulate hormones.

Oral contraceptives, anti-androgens, and insulin-sensitizing drugs are a few examples of medications that may be administered to treat particular symptoms and help the body achieve hormonal balance. Hormonal treatments, like drugs that induce ovulation,

may help women who want to get pregnant by improving their fertility and controlling their menstrual cycle.

Healthcare providers can assist in treating PCOS symptoms, control menstrual cycles, enhance fertility, and lower long-term health risks by reestablishing hormonal balance. Customizing treatment strategies for hormonal imbalances according to each patient's needs is crucial, taking into account the unique hormonal abnormalities that each PCOS woman has. Our understanding of the complex hormonal pathways behind PCOS is being deepened by ongoing research, which opens the door to more focused therapies aimed at improving patient outcomes.

In conclusion, hormonal imbalances—such as high testosterone, low progesterone, and elevated estrogen—are critical to the onset and progression of polycystic ovary syndrome (PCOS). These imbalances play a role in ovarian cyst formation, an ovulation, and irregular menstrual cycles.

Levels of Hormones and PCOS.

Recall that symptoms alone cannot be used to diagnose PCOS. An extremely complex endocrine condition is PCOS. Before a PCOS diagnosis is verified, comprehensive personal and family histories, an ultrasound to examine your reproductive organs, and blood tests to detect hormone levels should be performed. Your doctor will decide exactly which tests are required based on your symptoms. Hormone-level assessment has two main uses. Initially, it is helpful to rule out any other issues that could be the source of the symptoms. Secondly, it assists your doctor in confirming that you do indeed have PCOS in conjunction with an ultrasound and your personal and family histories. When evaluating a PCOS diagnosis, the following hormone levels are most frequently measured:

- hormone luteinizing (LH)
- The hormone that stimulates follicles (FSH)
- Complete and Unbound Testosterone
- DHEAS, or dehydroepiandrosterone sulfate
- lactating
- Forsoeveredione
- Gonadiene.

The following other hormones could be examined: Thyroid stimulating hormone (TSH), estrogen, and Moreover, tests for triglycerides, HDL, LDL, and cholesterol may be performed.

1. Follicle-stimulating hormone (FSH) and luteinizing hormone (LH).

The hormones that promote ovulation are LH and FSH. The brain's pituitary gland secretes both FSH and LH. LH and FSH levels at the start of the cycle typically vary from 5 to 20 ml/ml. LH and FSH levels in most women are roughly equal in the early stages of their cycles. But 24 hours before ovulation, there is an LH surge, during which the level of LH rises to roughly 25–40 ml/ml. The LH levels return to baseline after the ovary releases the egg.

Even though many PCOS-affected women still have FSH and LH levels in the 5–20 mlU/ml range, their LH levels are frequently two or three times higher than their FSH levels. For instance, LH levels of approximately 18 mlU/ml and FSH levels of approximately 6 mlU/ml are typical for women with PCOS (note that both values are within the normal range of 5–20 mlU/ml). This is regarded as a 3:1 ratio or an increased LH to FSH ratio. Ovulation can be interfered with by this shift in the LH to FSH ratio. Although this was once thought to be a crucial component in PCOS diagnosis, it is currently thought to be less helpful in diagnosing PCOS, but when considering the big picture, it's still beneficial.

Testimonials

Every female possesses testosterone in her body. Testosterone levels can be determined using two techniques:

Total Estrogen

No Cost Testosterone

The term "total testosterone" describes the entire concentration of all testosterone in your body, including free testosterone. This has a range of 6.0-86 ng/dl. The quantity of testosterone in your body that is free and functionally active is referred to as free testosterone. Typically, this quantity falls between 0.7 and 3.6 pg/ml. Total and free testosterone levels are frequently higher in PCOS-affected women. Furthermore, a woman's physiology can restrict natural ovulation and menstruation with even a small rise in testosterone.

2. S DHEA

All women contain the male hormone dehydroepiandrosterone or DHEA-S. The adrenal gland secretes an androgen called DHEA-S. DHEA-S levels in women are typically in the range of 35 to 430 ug/dl. The majority of PCOS-affected women often have DHEA-S levels higher than 200 ug/dl.

3. Lactating

A pituitary hormone called prolactin helps nursing moms produce and maintain milk. Women with PCOS typically have normal prolactin levels, which are less than 25 ng/ml. However, to rule out other issues, like a pituitary tumor, that could be producing PCOS-related symptoms, it's crucial to check for elevated prolactin levels. Prolactin levels are increased in some PCOS-affected women; they usually range from 25 to 40 ng/ml.

4. The hormone Androstenedione

The adrenal glands and ovaries both create the hormone ANDRO. Estrogen and testosterone levels can occasionally be impacted by elevated levels of this hormone. The range of normal ANDRO values is 0.7 – 3.1 ng/ml.

Testosterone

Following ovulation, the corpus luteum produces progesterone. The uterine lining becomes more receptive to progesterone during pregnancy. Progesterone levels are measured approximately 7 days after it is believed that ovulation has occurred in women with PCOS, particularly in those who are attempting to conceive through the use of fertility drugs. Progesterone levels above 14 ng/ml indicate that ovulation has taken place and the egg has been liberated from the ovary. Likely, the egg was not released if the progesterone level was low. This test is particularly crucial because, in certain cases, women with PCOS may exhibit symptoms of ovulation, but a progesterone test will reveal that ovulation has not taken place. If this occurs, your body might be creating a follicle and getting ready to ovulate, but the egg isn't coming out of the ovary for some reason. With the use of this information, your doctor may be able to modify your fertility prescription for the subsequent cycle to promote egg release.

Hormone

The hormone that is secreted by the ovaries and the adrenal glands in smaller amounts is called estrogen. Estradiol is the name of the most active form of estrogen in the body. Progesterone and estrogen must combine in an adequate proportion to initiate menstruation. The majority of PCOS-affected women are shocked to learn that their estrogen levels are within the normal range (about 25–75 pg/ml). This could be a result of the elevated insulin and testosterone levels that are occasionally converted to estrogen in PCOS-affected women.

SSH

The thyroid, a gland located in the neck, produces TSH, or thyroid stimulating hormone. TSH levels in PCOS-affected women typically range from 0.4 to 3.8 uIU/ml. To rule out other issues, such as an underactive or overactive thyroid, which frequently results in irregular or nonexistent periods and an ovulation, TSH is measured.

Sugar and Insulin.

In light of new evidence suggesting that insulin resistance is likely the root cause of PCOS, doctors are starting to consider glucose levels when making a diagnosis of PCOS. Depending on risk factors, the majority of women with polycystic ovary syndrome should undergo a glucose tolerance test and a fasting plasma glucose test at the time of diagnosis and then regularly after that. A high blood sugar level may be a sign of insulin resistance, a diabetes-related disorder that exacerbates polycystic ovary syndrome.

Heart Rate

When diagnosing and treating PCOS, some doctors may wish to check your cholesterol levels because research is starting to show a link between PCOS and heart disease. A significant risk factor for heart disease development is elevated cholesterol, which is more common in women with PCOS. The body often uses cholesterol, a material that resembles fat, to create hormones and cell membranes. A cholesterol level over 200 is regarded as high. Additionally, these levels may be evaluated since good (high-density lipoproteins, or HDL) and bad (low-density lipoproteins, or LDL) lipoprotein levels might sometimes be more suggestive of a woman's risk for developing heart disease.

An excessive amount of poor cholesterol tends to raise the risk of artery-clogging plaque, which can result in a heart attack. It is thought that having too much good cholesterol prevents cholesterol from accumulating in the arteries. Less good cholesterol and greater bad cholesterol are typically found in women with PCOS. Additionally, women with PCOS typically have high levels of triglycerides, another type of cholesterol, which raises their risk of heart disease. It's a good idea to have your cholesterol evaluated regularly even if your doctor does not check it when diagnosing PCOS because women with PCOS are more likely to acquire high cholesterol, which can result in heart disease.

Chapter 7

How Mental Health and PCOS Are Associated and What Can Be Done About It.

Your emotions and hormones are intertwined. This explains why mood fluctuations are a sign of postpartum depression in women, and why symptoms range from the baby blues to postpartum psychosis. Being a hormonal imbalance, polycystic ovary syndrome can also have a negative impact on your mental health. Here's how depression, PCOS, and other mental health conditions are related, along with some solutions.

The relationship between women's mental health disorders and PCOS

When women begin attempting to conceive and discover that they are having difficulties with their fertility, they are typically diagnosed with PCOS. Before your doctor orders testing to determine whether PCOS is present, you may go up to a year without getting pregnant. Even though PCOS may not be identified until later in life, many people are aware of its symptoms because they have been coping with it for a long time—often since they were teenagers.

Although irregular periods and facial hair are the primary physical signs of PCOS, many women are startled to learn that there is frequently a connection between PCOS and their emotional and mental health as well. Although women with PCOS may experience constant fatigue, reduced patience, and a decreased ability to handle stress, they frequently accept these symptoms as typical aspects of life. Although there has long been anecdotal evidence of a connection between PCOS and depression in women worldwide who experience the condition, the scientific community is only now beginning to catch up.

Although women with PCOS may experience constant fatigue, reduced patience, and a decreased ability to handle stress, they frequently accept these symptoms as typical aspects of life.

Researchers from Cardiff University's Neuroscience and Mental Health Research Institute found that women with PCOS have a higher likelihood of receiving a diagnosis for a variety of mental health issues. In order to progress toward a treatment plan and, ideally, a reduction in symptoms and an improvement in general quality of life, this provides individuals who are battling with PCOS and their mental health with a starting point for talking about the problem with their healthcare professionals.

Why does PCOS result in mental health issues?

More research is required to determine the precise cause and mechanism of PCOS's impact on mental health in relation to depression; however a number of its components are probably contributing causes. A hormone is the first. Hormone imbalances affect women with PCOS. This involves having too much testosterone and, occasionally, not enough progesterone, as well as having excess androgen hormones. All of this may result in severe and incapacitating anxiety, depression, impatience, and cognitive fog. Additionally, it may result in extreme mood swings, which may give off an air of unpredictability. In addition to feeling guilty for not managing life the way they believe they should, women who encounter these symptoms may also be embarrassed to discuss their struggles, which can exacerbate their anxiety and depressive symptoms.

PCOS's physical impacts may potentially be significant. In addition to excessive face and body hair, PCOS can result in thin, weak hair. It also makes weight loss challenging. All of this may result in problems with confidence and self-worth, which may then trigger eating disorders and depression. Infertility-related melancholy and anxiety can affect women who are trying to get pregnant but are having problems.

Which mental illnesses may be brought on by PCOS?

Depression and PCOS are associated with mood fluctuations, trouble getting out of bed, a breakdown in social interactions, and a lack of self-care. Nevertheless, a variety of additional mental health conditions, such as but not restricted to:

- Unease
- Manic episodes
- Severe depression conditions
- A bulimia
- Additional eating disorders

Somatizations: outward signs of unfavorable mental states

Personality sensibility

Since mental and physical health are related, it's critical to realize that having PCOS can put you at risk for mental health problems in addition to irregular periods.

Methods for treating PCOS-related mental health problems

Treatment options for PCOS-related mental health problems include managing the underlying PCOS as well as the mental health symptoms. Metformin is a medicine that is often prescribed to treat PCOS. It helps balance insulin and blood sugar levels, which can aid in weight loss and restore a more normal state of hormones. Women with PCOS have also benefited from concentrating on eating a nutritious, low-sugar diet and exercising frequently. To control their periods and address additional symptoms such as mood swings, acne, and excessive hair growth, PCOS patients may also use birth control.

There are two approaches to treating PCOS-related mental health issues:

- Addressing the underlying PCOS
- Treating the mental health symptoms individually.

The treatment of mental health disorders typically takes a multidisciplinary approach. Both talk therapy and cognitive behavioral therapy can be used to treat PCOS, anxiety episodes, depression associated with PCOS, and general concerns with self-esteem. Recording your emotions in a journal can assist you in identifying trends and stressors. You can also benefit from self-care and stress management techniques like massages, meditation, essential oil baths, or other practices that make you feel at ease and looked after.

When to visit a physician

It's crucial to look after your emotional and physical well-being, and you don't have to do it by yourself. Seeking treatment for depression, anxiety, PCOS, or any other mental health condition begins with a consultation with your physician.

It's time to visit a healthcare professional if any of the following symptoms are interfering with your everyday activities or giving you distress frequently or persistently:

- An overwhelming sense of dread or impending doom upon waking up and facing the day Oversleeping or napping Difficulty falling or remaining asleep
- Chronic self-doubt Difficulty taking pleasure in interpersonal connections
- Giving up interests or pastimes you used to love
- Being plagued by widespread anxiety
- A panic episode
- Unease

- Suicidal ideas or behaviors
- Even while anxiety, depression, and PCOS can coexist, mental health problems can also have other root causes. To properly treat your symptoms, you'll need to be certain that PCOS is the true source of your problems.

Get checked for PCOS, which typically entails blood tests and a basic ultrasound, if you are experiencing any of the following symptoms.

- Recent weight increase, especially in the abdominal area
- Inability to lose weight even with diet and exercise modifications
- Hair loss or thinning Excessive body and facial hair
- Irregular time frames
- Extended rounds lasting 35 days
- Extended or brief times
- Having trouble becoming pregnant
- Pregnancy errors

There is evidence linking PCOS to depression and other mental health problems, and you are not alone if you have been experiencing these symptoms. Although it's simple to assume that your symptoms are the result of life's everyday stresses, there might be therapies available to help you feel more like yourself and resume your regular activities. See your doctor about your symptoms and potential treatments if you're unsure if you have PCOS or whether it might be harming your mental health..

Chapter 8

PCOS treatment that is hormone-free.

One in ten women suffers from the hormonal condition known as polycystic ovarian syndrome, or PCOS. This is the most prevalent hormonal condition affecting fertile women. Symptoms such as irregular menstruation, infertility, weight gain, acne, and abnormal hair growth may result from it. Your doctor may suggest drugs that alter your insulin and hormone levels if you have PCOS. However, not everybody finds the thought of using prescription drugs appealing. Furthermore, a lot of people are hesitant to use long-term birth control.

The good news is that you may control your PCOS with natural treatment choices, ranging from lifestyle modifications to supplements.

Endocrinologist Dr. Carly Kelley of Duke Health states, "PCOS management is individualized." There isn't a "one-size-fits-all" solution or "cure." "Symptom management and the symptoms that are most important to each patient are the goals of treatment," she continues. Throughout the patient's lifetime, that could potentially alter.

Let's examine the most popular and efficacious alternative therapies for PCOS.

1. Bergamot

One substance that is taken from plants is berberine. In PCOS, berberine has been demonstrated to:

- An increase in pregnancy rates
- Boost your insulin resistance.
- Lower amounts of male sex hormone Lower levels of inflammation

Because berberine has an additive effect, several medical professionals advise using it with metformin or other diabetes drugs. This indicates that the drugs function better together than they would if taken alone.

2. Lead Zinc

A naturally occurring element, chromium aids in a few bodily metabolic processes. Certain grains are among the dietary sources of chromium that are poorly absorbed.

Chromium picolinate supplementation raises blood sugar and increases insulin sensitivity. Moreover, chromium promotes ovulation and aids in weight loss.

3. Xantopal

One B vitamin that can help reduce insulin resistance is thiol. In some PCOS situations, it has also been reported to aid with fertility.

You already have a chemical in your body called inositol. It facilitates insulin's ability to control blood sugar. There are nine distinct structures, or isomers, of isosorbide. In particular, it has been demonstrated that supplementing with Myo and D-chiro-Inositol in PCOS improves insulin resistance and hormone balance.

To reduce insulin resistance, regulate periods, and encourage ovulation and conception, women with PCOS who are looking for supplements or alternatives to traditional medical treatments might consider this, according to Dr. Kelley.

4. Probiotics as well as synbiotics

Good bacteria that aid in regulating gut function can be found in probiotics and synbiotics, which are a combination of prebiotics and probiotics. They also aid in controlling general inflammation. The balance of microorganisms in your stomach has an impact on insulin and glucose homeostasis, as well as body weight. These vitamins may aid in PCOS fertility and hormonal balance by lowering inflammation.

5. **Losing weight**

PCOS and weight have a complicated relationship. Researchers are unsure of whether PCOS causes weight gain or if elevated body fat causes PCOS. However, they are aware that controlling the symptoms and possible side effects of PCOS requires losing weight, exercising, and maintaining a balanced diet.

Gaining weight is associated with additional PCOS problems, including:

- Elevated blood pressure
- Headache
- Heart conditions
- Apnea in sleep
- Fatty liver illness

Thus, losing weight may benefit PCOS. Everybody's relationship with their body and weight is unique. If losing weight doesn't feel right for you, it doesn't have to be a health objective. It's interesting to note that exercise can raise ovulation and pregnancy rates in PCOS patients and improve insulin resistance, even in the absence of weight loss.

And a healthy diet can benefit you regardless of your weight objectives.

6. Nutrition

Some of the hormone abnormalities associated with PCOS may be mitigated by eating a balanced, healthful diet. It has not been demonstrated that any one diet is superior to another. Eating a comprehensive, well-balanced diet rich in nutrient-dense foods is essential.

Dr. Kelley advises consuming a diet strong in fiber and low in glycemic index. Fiber reduces the risk of insulin and blood sugar increases. Moreover, it facilitates digestion and raises satiety or the sensation of being full and content.

According to Kelley, "The best diet is generally the one you can stick to and sustain." She suggests eating a well-balanced diet reduced in processed foods, trans and saturated fats, and simple carbohydrates. It's also advised to have a diet high in fruits, vegetables, and lean proteins.

Managing your symptoms might be made easier if you eat the appropriate foods and stay away from particular ingredients. A healthy diet can aid in controlling your menstrual cycle and hormones. Consuming foods that have been excessively processed or stored can aggravate insulin resistance and inflammation.

Everything is about entire foods.

Preservatives, hormones, and artificial sweeteners are absent from whole foods. These foods are as near to their unadulterated, original state as can be achieved. Whole foods can be incorporated into your diet, such as fruits, vegetables, whole grains, and legumes.

Your body's endocrine system can more effectively control blood sugar levels if hormones and preservatives are absent.

Mix your protein and carbohydrate consumption.

Both protein and carbohydrates affect your hormone levels and level of energy. Consuming protein encourages the production of insulin in your body. High-carb, unprocessed foods Trusted Source may help increase insulin sensitivity. Rather than attempting a low-carb diet, concentrate on consuming adequate good protein.

The best Trusted Sources of protein are plant-based foods including healthy grains, legumes, and nuts.

Aim for anti-inflammatory PCOS, which is defined as low-level chronic inflammation in one study (Trusted Source). Including anti-inflammatory foods in your diet can assist in reducing your discomfort.

The Mediterranean diet is one option to think about. Inflammation is fought by olive oil, tomatoes, and leafy greens, fatty fish like tuna and mackerel, and tree nuts.

Increase your consumption of iron

Some PCOS-affected women bleed a lot when they get their period. Anemia or iron deficiency may arise from this. Discuss with your physician how you might increase your intake of iron if you have been diagnosed with either disease. They might advise you to increase your intake of iron-rich foods like broccoli, spinach, and eggs.

You should speak with your doctor before increasing your iron consumption. Iron overload can raise your risk Reliable Source of difficulties.

Increase your consumption of magnesium

Rich in magnesium and suitable for people with PCOS are almonds, cashews, spinach, and bananas.

Include some fiber to aid in digestion.

A high-fiber diet can aid in better digestion. Broccoli, Brussels sprouts, avocados, lima beans, lentils, and peas are all high in fiber.

Give up coffee.

There may be a connection between changes in estrogen levels, hormone behavior and caffeine usage. Consider using a decaf substitute, like an herbal tea, to increase your energy levels. The probiotic qualities of kombucha might also be advantageous.

If you're someone who needs their caffeine fix, try green tea. It has been demonstrated that green tea reduces insulin resistance Trusted Source. It can also support PCOS-afflicted women in controlling their weight.

7. Infusions

According to some studies, acupuncture may help PCOS patients ovulate more frequently. However, there isn't enough proof to say that acupuncture promotes fertility or ovulation at the moment.

Chapter 9

The PCOS diet:

How to control your PCOS with food

Many women suffer from polycystic ovarian syndrome, however dietary and lifestyle modifications can significantly lessen symptoms. A licensed dietitian defines a PCOS diet in this context.

You may be familiar with the abbreviation PCOS, but you may not be entirely sure what it means. It is an acronym for polycystic ovary syndrome, an endocrine condition affecting those born with a female chromosome. Though the precise inheritance rate—roughly 70%—is unknown, it is thought to be inherited genetically.

Although PCOS can be a frustrating illness that affects your menstrual cycle, fertility, weight, and looks, most people with the disorder can live normal, healthy lives with the help of healthcare specialists and lifestyle modifications. This includes managing some of your symptoms by adhering to a PCOS diet.

Who is affected by PCOS, what is it, and why?

First things first, let's define PCOS. The condition known as polycystic ovarian syndrome can lead to issues with our reproductive system, metabolism, and hormones. Because it affects the endocrine system, which is the body's hormone regulation system, this is the reason it is referred to as an endocrine condition in scientific terminology.

Despite the name, PCOS is not exclusive to people with polycystic ovaries," says registered dietician and PCOS specialist Lauren Talbert. She clarifies that this is a common misperception about the condition, as PCOS can occur in people without ovarian cysts. All it takes to receive a PCOS diagnosis is two of the following conditions:

Several ovarian cysts. Your healthcare provider can use an ultrasound to identify them.

An irregular menstrual cycle is defined as less than nine monthly periods more than thirty-five days between periods, or missing periods or ovulation.

high concentrations of androgen hormones also referred to as masculine hormones. Usually, your healthcare professional can identify this through laboratory testing, but occasionally, physical symptoms can also aid in the diagnosing process.

According to Talbert, "the cause of PCOS is still not fully known." There is a theory that states it is triggered by environmental circumstances and inherited genetically. However because many individuals with PCOS also have insulin resistance, scientific study has come to attribute it more and more to this condition. Insulin is a hormone that controls the movement of glucose from the bloodstream into the cells, which helps lower blood sugar levels. Your body isn't doing this process correctly if you have insulin resistance, which results in an excess of sugar in your system.

According to Talbert, the most prevalent indicator of PCOS is an irregular menstrual cycle, with some individuals experiencing months or even years without a monthly cycle.

PCOS diet: What dietary and lifestyle choices can you make to help control PCOS?

"The main strategies for managing PCOS are diet and lifestyle," states Talbert. Because diet and health are frequently related. According to Talbert, the main strategies for managing PCOS are diet and lifestyle. This is because food and reproductive health are frequently related. "Remember that a lifestyle that combats insulin resistance is most beneficial, as it is a key component of this condition."

But it's critical to distinguish at this stage. According to Talbert, "another misconception is that all women with PCOS are overweight or obese." According to research, between 40% and 80% of PCOS sufferers are overweight or obese, but they are all at risk for metabolic problems. This implies that your body's capacity to turn food and liquids into energy may nonetheless be a touch-off regardless of your weight. For instance, compared to individuals without PCOS, those with PCOS typically have greater cholesterol and more fat in their organs.

Therefore, losing weight can help with menstrual cycle regulation and insulin sensitivity. This Australian study demonstrated that reducing body weight by as little as 5% to 10% could help with PCOS symptoms. Nevertheless, anyone suffering from PCOS would probably benefit from a few dietary and lifestyle adjustments.

PCOS diet: foods to eat and foods to avoid

According to Talbert, the majority of studies conducted to date have backed up three main diets that are said to help with PCOS symptoms: the Mediterranean diet, the DASH diet (Dietary Approach to Stop Hypertension), and a low-glycemic index diet. All three of these strategies can assist people with PCOS in losing weight and reducing inflammation, according to research.

According to Talbert, "All of these diets are high in fiber, which has been shown to improve insulin resistance." As Talbert points out, they are also typically high in plant-based foods like nuts, seeds, legumes, and whole grains as well as a variety of healthful unsaturated fats like olive oil, nuts, seeds, and fatty fish (like salmon).

Simple methods to stick to a PCOS diet plan

Finding out more about these diets is a terrific place to start, but you're not required to follow them precisely. It is simple to begin by implementing a few minor adjustments to your daily diet. This could entail increasing the amount of fruit, vegetables, whole grains, legumes, nuts, seeds, and lean protein—like chicken and fish—that you use in your meals, along with olive oil.

Our nutritionist advises getting started easily:

- Replace processed grains with whole grains.
- During meals, include one or two servings of fruit or vegetables.
- Consume some nuts.
- Switch out the red meat with fish.

Avoid foods like red meat, fried foods, creamy sauces, desserts, and sugary drinks that are high in saturated fat and/or sugar.

You can also begin by substituting plant-based protein for red meat in your diet. For example, try black bean burgers or lentil soup in place of beef chili. Or try coming up with creative methods to eat more fruits and vegetables. Maybe making cauliflower rice or spiralizing veggies instead of spaghetti might be better choices for you. Other simple substitutions include shifting to a veggie and dip snack rather than chips.

Conclusion:

Treatment Trends and Prevention

Why is awareness of PCOS important?
PCOS is receiving more attention than it has in the past due to initiatives like Polycystic Ovary Awareness Month. According to Dr. Tahir Mahmood, "surveys of women have suggested that PCOS is underdiagnosed." Many women suffer from worry as a result of their inadequate knowledge about PCOS. People are frequently diagnosed with PCOS as well.
early in life, while their bodies are still developing physiologically.

Additionally, he claims that many practitioners lack experience in managing young teens who worry about their appearance, may have some acne, and are quite self-conscious about their irregular periods. These physicians frequently diagnose teenagers with PCOS and provide a prescription for birth control tablets.
In reality, though, a diagnosis has not been made. Nothing has been tested. And it starts to feel like a shame in their lives that they might not even have

PCOS, even though they may have it, says Dr. Mahmood According to recent worldwide guidelines on PCOS, a diagnosis of PCOS should be made eight years after menarche.

Quote from Tahir Mahmood" He adds that it's still unclear why some individuals get PCOS and others don't, as well as why certain racial groups are more likely to get it. We refer to it as a multi factorial condition because, in addition to genetic and racial predispositions, environmental variables also play a significant role. The body mass index, or average BMI, is rising globally and is more pronounced in some populations than others.

As per Dr. Mahmood, a greater grasp of the true nature of PCOS is necessary. However, he claims that the primary problem is that people view it as a sickness. It is a syndrome rather than an illness, with a range of symptoms, aberrant metabolic processes, and variable clinical presentations. Above all, there is still no accepted method for reaching a verified diagnosis.

What are the risk factors for PCOS?

PCOS has trigger factors in addition to the previously listed risk factors, which include genetics and environment. But a high body mass index is the most significant one, according to Dr. Mahmood (BMI).

PCOS can be identified by Ultrasonography in up to 15% of women with normal BMIs. Not every person with a high BMI will exhibit every symptom of PCOS and will likely experience regular cycles. Women in Northern Europe, Southeast Asia, and even Southern Europe differ from one another when it comes to the high BMI symptoms of PCOS.

One significant issue that is frequently discussed is whether obesity causes PCOS or PCOS causes obesity.

There are many risk factors associated with PCOS in addition to genetics and environment. A high body mass index, however, is the most significant (BMI).

According to Dr. Mahmood, "It's crucial to keep in mind that insulin insensitivity is a major factor in the manifestation of PCOS symptoms." We're trying to figure out why there are racial variations in the symptoms that people experience, such as irregular periods and facial hair growth, once their BMI begins to rise.

Moreover, he claims that environmental influences are also quite important. Water pollution from increased chemical use in agriculture and industry directly affects the development of sperm, eggs, and progeny.

A major contributing element to the onset of PCOS symptoms is insulin insensitivity.

Thus, there are several variables that we are discovering more and more. New studies attempting to explain why some women have these symptoms while others do not are published almost daily.

People today start having periods earlier than they used to, due to a variety of other causes. For example, it's not unusual for someone to begin having periods at the age of 10 or 11. Dr. Mahmood clarifies that body fat is one of the factors. Therefore, menarche occurs earlier in those who have greater adolescent body fat. There is a subset of individuals who experience a delayed onset of menstruation, occurring beyond the age of 16, for which there is no known medical explanation.

How does PCOS feel on the body?

Period irregularities and excessive hair development, which can appear as facial hair (typically on the chin, upper lip, and occasionally as sideburns), are the most common signs of PCOS. Additionally, it may result in hair growth beneath the belly button and around the nipples.

Some PCOS sufferers develop face acne. It can range in intensity from moderate to severe (dark-headed pimples), and it depends on the genetic group. According to Dr. Mahmood, young ladies from Southeast Asia and possibly even Southern Europe are more likely to suffer from that kind of illness.

Excessive facial hair and acne can affect some people's confidence levels," states Dr. Mahmood. Some people may have infertility, which can lead to depression in those who are attempting to conceive. Usually, this call for additional research and care from an infertility specialist. Furthermore, some PCOS patients may experience unfavorable pregnancy outcomes, like hypertension and gestational diabetes, if they do become pregnant. Naturally, the majority of these ladies want something to be done about it.

How is PCOS diagnosed by medical professionals?

Dr. Mahmood claims that there is a great deal of dispute in this field. After diagnosing a patient with clinical characteristics such as irregular periods, increased body hair growth, or acne, most doctors order blood testing.

"In a perfect world, consideration should be given to the patient's age and unique characteristics, as well as their weight and any clinical manifestations (as previously mentioned). Hormonal testing should come last."

According to him, it's crucial to avoid taking random blood samples for hormonal testing at any random point during a cycle because different menstrual cycles have different phases with varying hormone levels. Doing them during a period during the early follicular phase is preferred. Although measuring free testosterone is preferable, not everyone will have elevated levels. According to most research, 60 percent of women will have higher testosterone levels.

Finding the free androgen index, a ratio that assesses aberrant androgen (male hormone) levels, is another helpful test.

According to Dr. Mahmood, pelvic Ultrasonography scans might occasionally display the telltale signs of PCOS while the ovaries seem normal.

Therefore, in addition to using blood tests and ultrasound scans, the clinician should also consider the clinical signs while making a diagnosis. Before diagnosing someone with PCOS, it's crucial to consider their age because physiological changes in their youth may cause irregular cycles.

In conclusion, there isn't a single, ideal method for PCOS diagnosis.

How should medical professionals handle treating PCOS patients?

According to Dr. Tahir Mahmood, education is the key to raising awareness of the disease and how it affects one's self-confidence. Young people should be treated with more empathy, and their concerns should be taken seriously the specialist's education is significant in that regard as well.

According to Dr. Mahmood, specialty and family medicine training differs globally.

People are especially taught more about and have a better awareness of endocrine disorders in certain nations. These specialists have received less specialized training in other nations, and some may not have received training covering all facets of women's health.

He adds that the majority of medical professionals mainly focus on endocrine issues. They might be experts in treating problems related to pregnancy, cancer, bladder troubles, and fertility, but they might not have received the necessary training to handle women with endocrine disorders, which is where PCOS comes in.

Approximately 8–13 percent of people with PCOS, making it a sizable community. However, not every provider of women's health has the same level of proficiency in identifying the most effective PCOS treatment.

Which PCOS signs are essential to monitor to get an early diagnosis and potentially avoid the condition?

Dr. Mahmood offers several recommendations for identifying and avoiding PCOS symptoms in their early stages.

1. **Maintain a period log**

If your menstruation is irregular, the first thing you should do is keep a diary. The days that the menstrual cycle begins and ends should be noted in the diary with clarity. Keep this journal for six to twelve months. It will be helpful to have this record when you see a professional. According to Dr. Mahmood although they don't occur every four weeks, it's possible from the diary that periods are occurring every five to six weeks, which is typical for that age group. Especially for girls under the age of eighteen."

2. **Recognize when to perform a pelvic Ultrasonography**

A common question is whether a young adult with PCOS needs to be referred for a pelvic ultrasound scan. According to Dr. Mahmood, the most recent international guidelines regarding PCOS state that, "at least before eight years have elapsed from the onset of periods, the diagnosis of PCOS should not be made by ultrasound scan."

Therefore, he recommends waiting until age 19 to perform an ultrasound scan to identify PCOS in someone who begins having periods at age 11. This is crucial since early adolescence's growing hypothalamus-pituitary-ovarian axis maturation process and pubertal development share similarities that could lead to confusion with PCOS. Mahmood asserts, "It is the clinician's duty to inform the patient and their parents about the ongoing maturation of their hormonal systems

3. **Keep an eye on your calories.**

Eating low-glycemic foods is advised by Dr. Mahmood, particularly fruits and vegetables. By doing this, the chance of accumulating extra fat around the waist can be decreased. We observe it every day: according to reports, the average waist size is increasing. Exercise regularly can help prevent waist enlargement. It has been shown that people with a waist-hip ratio (WRH) of more than one may be at longer risk of acquiring various conditions over time, including diabetes and hypertension.

A healthy BMI often falls between 18.5 and 25. Furthermore, the menstrual cycle may become erratic after it reaches 30, which is thought to be an indication of PCOS, according to Dr. Mahmood.

Diet for PCOS therapy

According to Tahir Mahmood, diet is essential because controlling weight is a lifestyle strategy. Additionally, every management situation is unique; there is no quick fix.

Dr. Mahmood asserts that low-glycemic diets and foods high in antioxidants are beneficial. Data on the DASH (Dietary Approaches to Stop Hypertension) dietary plan, which primarily consists of consuming low-sodium and well-balanced foods, has just been released. It has been demonstrated that DASH reduces free glucose levels, which causes insulin to be released.

According to Dr. Mahmood, dietary supplements can also be beneficial. One particular food supplement called inositol is said to have favorable effects on the hormonal profile of PCOS. Its efficacy in young people requires further study.

Regular exercise is advised for up to 150 minutes a week, 90 minutes of moderate-to-intense activity, and so on, according to Dr. Mahmood.

Medicines and prescriptions

Prescriptions ought to be written based on symptoms, according to Dr. Mahmood. According to him, birth control tablets are a safe option for a young person who does not smoke and whose BMI is under thirty if the primary symptom is irregular cycles.

Deep vein thrombosis is a risk factor for those using birth control pills whose BMI is more than thirty, and that risk rises as the BMI rises above thirty-five. Therefore, it's critical to select a prescription that can lower the risk and consider this.

Dr. Mahmood states, "Metformin is a medication that is frequently used for Type 2 diabetes. However, this medication improves insulin insensitivity, a condition that is frequently present in obese and PCOS patients alike. Although the medication is commonly used, it's crucial to talk to your endocrinologist about it before taking it.

Dr. Mahmood notes that there isn't a rapid cure for hirsutism, or excessive facial hair development, which is a side effect of PCOS. Most hormone therapy for this lasts between 12 and 18 months. Because free testosterone promotes hair growth, the goal of hormonal medications is to reduce it. Doctors occasionally recommend non-hormonal diuretics that can reduce the amount of free testosterone in the body. If they are prescribed, the doctor must monitor electrolytes and liver function.

If they so choose, people can also think about non-medical options like laser treatment and waxing," advises Dr. Mahmood. If someone also takes weight control plans into consideration, their potential benefits may be amplified. While the intensity of hair growth may lessen, none of these therapies have a lasting effect. Certain anti-androgen lotions can also be used to treat facial hair development.

Because every medicine has the potential to create side effects, it's crucial to talk with your healthcare professional about customized treatment alternatives.

Does PCOS improve after bariatric surgery?

According to Dr. Mahmood, bariatric surgery has very little use in the treatment of PCOS. Although bariatric surgery reduces weight, it also affects how well nutrients are absorbed. It won't immediately reduce hirsutism, even if it will decrease free testosterone levels. Overall, it can lead to a positive trend of biochemical changes in the person, and if they have sufficiently shed pounds, it may also greatly improve the regularity of their menstrual cycle. But neither PCOS nor hirsutism can be cured by it.

Can PCOS be cured with homeopathy?

Dr. Mahmood states, "We have no experience using homeopathy." Furthermore, no extensive research has been done to demonstrate its advantages over conventional medications that are routinely prescribed. Contrary to what proponents of homeopathy claim, there is no miracle treatment for PCOS.

Does yoga aid with PCOS management?

According to Dr. Mahmood, yoga helps reduce anxiety and enhance mood. Though yoga can assist individuals in managing their emotions and symptoms more positively, it is not a natural remedy for PCOS.

Has anyone ever fully recovered from PCOS?

Not really, Dr. Mahmood responds. Once PCOS has shown symptoms, there is no complete cure. The severity of PCOS symptoms can only be decreased.

According to Dr. Mahmood, an ovary that has undergone polycystic development will continue to do so. However effective management makes the manifestation less obvious.

Once PCOS has shown symptoms, there is no complete cure. There is only so much that can be done to lessen PCOS symptoms.

For instance, there's a higher than 80% likelihood that a person's periods will become regular if they manage to aggressively lose weight and lower their BMI from 35 to 25. Their acne is more likely to clear up, and they might not need to take antibiotics or hormone therapy. Additionally, their hirsutism will improve. However, the ovarian alteration that has occurred will not go away. Therefore, if an ultrasound scan is performed, the diagnosis of polycystic ovary would still be made.

What occurs if PCOS is not managed?

According to Dr. Mahmood, there is no research on the normal course of PCOS in any racial or weight category.

"We need to consider the person's age and BMI. It won't make much of a difference if a person with irregular cycles and a BMI under 25 is found to have PCOS by scanning. It won't change, he promises. On the other hand, a person with a BMI of 35 who has irregular periods, PCOS on an ultrasound exam, and inadequate weight management is more likely to develop metabolic syndrome. The lifetime chance of developing Type 2 diabetes and the related cardiovascular hazards is elevated in those with metabolic syndrome.

Additionally, according to Dr. Mahmood, a woman with PCOS and a higher BMI who gets pregnant runs the risk of developing gestational diabetes, which can be harmful to both her and the unborn child. If they don't drop a sizable amount of weight after giving birth, over 40% of pregnant women with gestational diabetes will get Type 2 diabetes seven years after the pregnancy.

According to Dr. Mahmood, cardiovascular disease is another concern.

"PCOS is a risk factor, but there are many other variables at play when heart disease develops. Depending on the person in question—do they smoke? Do they suffer from any other illnesses, such as hypertension or a metabolic issue related to cholesterol? Are their thyroid glands underactive? Many patients with PCOS may also have additional health issues. When it comes to PCOS sufferers, all of these variables significantly raise their chance of having heart disease.

How to lessen PCOS-related facial hair development

According to Dr. Mahmood, the degree of hirsutism determines how it should be treated.

1. First, it's important to ascertain whether PCOS is the only cause of hirsutism. Other endocrine glands besides the ovaries might also intensify

hirsutism. To ensure that the diagnosis of PCOS is accurate, the thyroid and adrenal glands should also be examined at the initial examination, and blood tests should be performed.

2. Secondly, hair growth will be quantifiably impacted by any PCOS treatment that reduces free testosterone and free androgen levels. The hair condition known as hirsutism has a protracted lifespan. Before any hair grows on the skin, it takes six to nine months to develop. Given that hair follicles continue to form, any treatment must be administered for a considerable amount of time—ideally, 12 to 18 months—and may even be lifelong.

Dr. Mahmood continues by saying that laser ablation of hair follicles is an option for those who would rather not receive hormonal treatment. A greater effect on hair regrowth is achieved with this concentrated laser treatment than with medicine alone since it destroys the base of the hair follicles. But not every laser works the same way, and some people react negatively to them on their skin.

He claims that because various persons react differently to different laser preparations, laser treatment does not provide permanent outcomes.

Certain racial groups cannot benefit from certain laser modalities, and certain locations require highly specialized laser preparations. A single, targeted laser may be effective in treating thick hair growth, but not many. Therefore, the optimal laser for this individual needs to be determined by the doctor or beautician.

3. Dr. Mahmood wants to emphasize weight control in his third point. It's critical to strive toward a

 BMI under 25, as this will lower the blood levels of free testosterone.

Is PCOS a possible cause of hair loss?

According to Dr. Mahmood, any endocrine disorders with elevated amounts of androgens in the blood can result in widespread thinning of scalp hair, which, in severe cases, can cause considerable scalp hair loss.

Dr. Mahmood lists several potential illnesses and reasons why people may lose hair:

Disorders like PCOS and those that impact the adrenal gland (Cushing syndrome, congenital adrenal hyperplasia)

Long-term illnesses (such as diabetes, lupus, inflammatory bowel disease, liver disease, iron insufficiency, and, in rare cases, syphilis) and underactive thyroid

Usage of medications (chemotherapy, carbimazole, anabolic steroids, anticoagulants, antidepressants, and oral contraceptives)

Excessive dieting, inadequate protein consumption, and poor nutrition

The susceptibility of hair follicles to the hormone DHT (dihydrotestosterone)

Age Genetics (occurs in postmenopausal years occasionally)

Because there are so many possible causes, Dr. Mahmood believes it's important to be evaluated by a professional with significant knowledge in endocrinology, not just an interest in PCOS.

What advice would you provide to transgender and non-conforming individuals with PCOS?

The effects of PCOS can be masculinizing, which some people may find appealing. They would like to develop a mustache, for example.

According to Dr. Mahmood, individuals are free to live however they like. "Medicine must take into account the needs of the patient and how it can best support them."

He feels it boils down to personal preference. However, it's equally critical to recognize that high levels of male-type hormones might negatively impact lipid profiles. The lipid profile, which includes metabolites of fat and cholesterol, raises the risk of cardiovascular disease, thus treatment strategies must take it into account.

What recent developments exist in PCOS research?

According to Dr. Mahmood, research is progressing in determining the most effective means of diagnosing and treating PCOS and its different forms.

Second, he claims that research is shifting toward a more targeted strategy for treating patients with a range of manifestations since some of them may have very few symptoms or even PCOS with cycle issues, which calls for an alternative course of care.

According to Dr. Mahmood, "There is then a group of people who have severe manifestations of the condition." By utilizing natural and low-glycemic dietary supplements, we are attempting to comprehend how to control hormonal treatment. The encouragement of a healthy lifestyle and a lifecycle approach are the new focal points. A sizable contingent of specialists favors educating individuals about PCOS as opposed to overmedicating them with hormones.

Additionally, he states that the use of laser therapy for hair growth is expanding quickly and that we must find out which kind of laser is most effective for treating particular forms of hirsutism as well as the long-term effects of these therapies on hair regrowth.

Excessive hair loss from PCOS can result in baldness and widespread hair thinning. More investigation is required into local therapies, medications that bind to free circulating androgens, and the contribution of anti-inflammatory and hair growth stimulants to hair loss.

Of course, bariatric surgery is becoming more and more popular, as it can assist individuals in managing their weight and leading healthier lives.

Lastly, Mahmood asserts, "We must make a greater effort to understand women's needs and desires, as well as the effects of their circumstances on them. Furthermore, we now understand that PCOS significantly affects both energy and mental health. Psychiatrists are contributing more and more as a means of understanding how to help PCOS sufferers instead of trying to uncover a miracle treatment.

Advice from Dr. Mahmood to those suffering from PCOS

In addition to having reasonable expectations and having a realistic conversation, it's critical to encourage patients to ask their doctors tough questions during examinations and visits. Dr. Mahmood says. Talking about your symptoms, the tests you need, and your exact diagnosis is a realistic conversation.

It is also important to anticipate that the doctor might not always have all the answers. PCOS is no known cure, thus each patient needs to locate a qualified expert who can take care of them and be patient. Tahir Mahmood claims that the condition is permanent.

It's not cancerous. It's not an illness. It is a syndrome with a variety of symptoms that present in various ways. Additionally, each ailment needs to be managed; therefore they should collaborate closely with their doctor.

Finally, returning to my most popular lifestyle intervention, I would advise you to maintain a low blood sugar level by eating a diet high in antioxidant-rich, low-glycemic foods and drinking lots of non-fizzy fluids. Eat three meals a day and break the habit of buying food at a fast-food restaurant whenever you feel peckish.